Linguistics for Language Teachers

This book is an accessible introduction to linguistics specifically tailored for teachers of second language/bilingual education. It guides teachers stepwise through the components of language, focusing on the areas of linguistics that are most pertinent for teaching. Throughout the book there are opportunities to analyze linguistic data and discuss language-related issues in various educational and social contexts. Readers will be able to identify patterns in actual language use to inform their teaching and help learners advance to the next level. A highly readable account of how language works, this book is an ideal text for teacher education courses.

Sunny K. Park-Johnson is an assistant professor in the College of Education at DePaul University. She received her Ph.D. in linguistics from Purdue University. Park-Johnson directs the Bilingual-Bicultural Education Minor and co-directs the Bilingual Language Development Lab. Her research interests include bilingual and heritage language development and maintenance, morphosyntax, and the intersection of theoretical linguistics, applied linguistics, and education.

Sarah J. Shin is Associate Provost for Academic Affairs at the University of Maryland Baltimore County, where she is also a professor of education. She received her Ph.D. in linguistics from the University of Michigan and specializes in bilingualism, heritage language education, and TESOL teacher preparation. Shin is the author of *Bilingualism in schools and society* (Routledge, 2018), *English language teaching as a second career* (Multilingual Matters, 2017), and *Developing in two languages* (Multilingual Matters, 2005).

Linguistics for Language Teachers

Lessons for Classroom Practice

**Sunny K. Park-Johnson
and Sarah J. Shin**

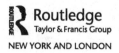

NEW YORK AND LONDON

First published 2020
by Routledge
52 Vanderbilt Avenue, New York, NY 10017

and by Routledge
2 Park Square, Milton Park, Abingdon, Oxon, OX14 4RN

Routledge is an imprint of the Taylor & Francis Group, an informa business

© 2020 Taylor & Francis

Library of Congress Cataloging-in-Publication Data
A catalog record for this book has been requested

ISBN: 978-1-138-68182-8 (hbk)
ISBN: 978-1-138-68193-4 (pbk)
ISBN: 978-1-315-54546-2 (ebk)

Typeset in Times New Roman
by Apex CoVantage LLC

(Sunny's dedication)
For Drew, Raela, and Vinny

(Sarah's dedication)
For Ron Schwartz and Jodi Crandall

Contents

Tables

Figures

Acknowledgments

We would like to thank all the people who have helped us in writing this book. We thank our editors at Routledge, Ze'ev Sudry and Helena Parkinson, for their guidance and support throughout the process. We also want to express our gratitude to the reviewers for their insightful feedback.

Sunny would like to thank her wonderful colleagues at DePaul University for their support, especially Sonia Soltero and Jason Goulah. She also thanks her former professors, particularly Elena Benedicto, Elaine Francis, and Mary Niepokuj, who instilled the love of language, linguistics, and sharing it through teaching, and to her parents and brother for creating a linguistically diverse home. Sunny also wishes to thank her many multilingual friends, colleagues, and RAs who helped come up with examples from many different languages. She also owes so much to her coauthor, Sarah, for the opportunity and mentorship. Finally, Sunny is deeply grateful for her husband Andrew and their children Raela and Vinny for providing infinite love, laughter, and groundedness.

Sarah is grateful for the enduring support of her colleagues at the University of Maryland Baltimore County, especially Mary Tabaa, Jiyoon Lee, and Doaa Rashed. She dedicates this book to Ron Schwartz and Jodi Crandall, who invited her to join the UMBC TESOL program in 1999 and have been her steadfast champions ever since. The students in Sarah's linguistics course over the years have been instrumental in helping her envision this book. Her students remain a constant source of inspiration, and she hopes this book will help practitioners like them for years to come. Finally, Sarah wishes to thank her coauthor, Sunny, for doing this book with her. A talented collaborator who can both complement and expand one's thinking is every scholar's dream, and Sunny is exactly that.

Acknowledgments

1 The Components of Language

1.1 Introduction

What do you know when you know a language?

Many people may say that when you know a language, you can communicate a message or perhaps hold a conversation in the language. You might be able to exchange information, greet someone, ask someone for directions, read a menu, or write a letter. These are certainly important language functions and tasks that we want our students to learn—and you might feel like you know the language when you can accomplish these tasks—but it still doesn't quite describe what language is. To use an analogy, we know the human body has important functions for survival, like breathing, blood circulation, and digestion. However, these functions do not exactly describe *what* the human body consists of or how it uses its components to accomplish those tasks. Similarly, to answer the question *What do you know when you know a language?*, we need to know what language consists of and how it uses its components to accomplish language functions. That's where linguistics steps in.

Linguistics is the scientific study of language. Linguists aim to look at language objectively, observing how it functions "in the wild", how it grows, how it changes, and how it is used. Language is studied scientifically like any natural phenomenon, as a botanist would study a plant or a microbiologist would study bacteria. This is different from what grammar books sometimes do, which is to prescribe how it *should* be used and what constitutes proper language. Linguists analyze language for what it is and how it is actually used by its speakers. They study everything from the smallest components (e.g., how much air is needed to make a /p/ sound like a /p/) to the largest components (e.g., how people apologize politely in text messages). They study everyone from newborn babies to elderly people. They study spoken and signed languages. They study languages spoken by billions of people and languages spoken by ten people. They study how language changes over hundreds of years and how language changes over a couple of months. They study languages with social power and languages that are forbidden and spoken in secret. There are entire books written on the syntax and pragmatics of profanity. The sky's the limit.

1.2 Linguistics and Language Teachers

Language teachers are linguists. While you may believe that teaching students how to speak a language is a different job description than analyzing language, the two are inextricably linked. In order to develop the best way to approach a new lesson, address a pattern of errors across a student's work, or explain a concept in the target language that simply does not exist in the students' first language, teachers have to first identify and understand the inner workings of the language. A doctor would not begin a treatment without understanding how the human body works; a mechanic would not begin to fix a car without understanding how the machinery functions. It's important for language teachers to be able to recognize and understand the parts, as well as the relationships between those parts.

Related to this, language teachers are more than just users of the language themselves. Simply being able to speak the language does not mean you can necessarily teach it; we certainly would not expect that someone can be a doctor simply because they have been sick before, or that they can be a mechanic because they drive a car regularly. To teach a language, it's helpful to not only be able to speak the language but understand what it is you are using when you speak it. Additionally, if you are to be a language teacher, you need to know how to analyze and consider language metalinguistically. When students ask you "why is it X but not Y?" and if your answer to their question is, "I don't know, that's just how it is", then they're not learning much from the experience. Or, if a student in your class makes the same error time after time, it's not enough that we say, "let's practice not making that error". The language teacher has to identify the error and recognize the pattern of occurrence. That's a main part of what linguistics is: patterns and tendencies and characteristics of language. But we don't stop there. Not only is it important for teachers to recognize the pattern, but then try to explain it. That is where linguistics—and specifically linguistic theories—comes into play. Theories help us make sense of what is going on with our students, and from there we have solutions that we can bring back to the classroom. Language teachers are linguists because they need to be aware of what is going on in the language they speak and teach, analyze these patterns, and make sense of them.

However, there is a problem. Linguists are trained to do these things, but language teachers are not. This is a grave error and a gap in our teacher training. Much of the focus of language teacher training is on methods and the teacher's own language proficiency, both of which are certainly important and necessary. However, language teachers do not receive much linguistics training; they are not often explicitly taught the structure of their language, or how to analyze linguistic data. Consequently, being less knowledgeable about the target language means teachers often rely on the textbook to learn about the language, which takes away from the autonomy of the teacher. Many language teacher candidates have sheepishly confessed that they "don't really get grammar" or that they feel intimidated by linguistics and wished it was part of their training.

Language teachers also benefit from linguistics training because there is an entire world of research and resources out there about language acquisition, bilingualism, heritage languages, classroom language learning, and how the specifics of your target language work (e.g., how German speakers determine which pronoun to use to mean *you*, what sound changes are occurring in contemporary Quechua). The problem is, these academic sources are written for linguists, not practitioners. Like many scientific fields, linguistics has a complex set of jargon that is not transparent for the majority of the population, even language teachers who really have an invested interest in language. Theta roles, sister nodes, and voiceless alveolar fricatives have no meaning for people outside of the linguistic subfields. Not to mention the array of acronyms that we must muddle through: NOM, ACC, NP, VP. Accessibility for teachers means that when they read a linguistics article, book, or academic resource, they can understand what they mean and use these resources to expand their knowledge base. It is not acceptable that language teachers are simply cut off from these resources that can help them continue to learn or to find helpful guidance about a particular aspect of the language they are teaching (or the language(s) their students are coming to school with). Are teachers supposed to twiddle their thumbs and wait for an "easy-to-read" version of the research—which could take years—or should teachers be given the tools and skills from the start so they can access the latest, most up-to-date research and resources? We will let you guess what we think.

1.3 The Layers

Language consists of multiple layers, much like a layered cake. Each layer serves an important function, but to get the full experience, you need all of these components in order for a language to be a language. When you serve a piece of cake, you slice your knife downward so that you get a little of every layer. Language works the same way: when you know a language, you have to know a portion of all of those layers. Let's inspect each layer briefly here.

The first layer is phonetics, which is the smallest unit of language. **Phonetics** is the study of the sounds of languages, which come together to form syllables, words, phrases, sentences, and paragraphs. It is analogous to the cells in our bodies: they are the building blocks. Every language and dialect has a unique set of sounds, or **phonetic inventory**, that is used to build the language. As language teachers and learners, we know that there are sounds in the target language that might be different from the languages we already know, and one of the many challenges is to learn how to make these sounds that are new to us. Perhaps you have struggled with rolling your *r* sounds when learning Spanish or making the *th* sound in English, as in the word *think*. What can be even more difficult is learning how to hear and distinguish sounds that are not in the languages you speak, like the distinction between *tal* (moon), *ttal* (daughter), and *tʰal* (mask) in Korean, which is very difficult to distinguish if you are a native English speaker. This is because we tend to hear and produce sounds that are most familiar to us. Another important aspect of phonetics is the acoustics of sound, like pitch, length, or amplitude, which can change how we hear the sound. Thus, knowing the phonetics layer of a language means you know how to use, hear, and differentiate sounds in the language.

The next layer of the language cake is **phonology**. Many people use phonology interchangeably with phonetics, but there is an important distinction. While phonetics is the study of sounds, phonology is the study of the relationship between these sounds. For example, think of a string of numbers as in a phone number: 754–6794. When you say each individual number in isolation, it will sound like it does in (1). But when you say the numbers together in a string, which is what most people do, you glide from one sound to another. Some of the sounds even change. See (2).

(1) *seven five four, six seven nine four*
(2) *sevem fife four, sik seven nime four*

You will notice that when you say the string of numbers naturally at normal speed, the /n/ in *seven* changes to something that sounds more like /m/ before the /f/ in *five*, so that you end up saying *sevem* instead of *seven*. Similarly, the /n/ in *nine* changes to /m/ before /f/ in *four*, so it sounds more like *nime* than *nine*. These changes occur to make the transition from one number to the next sound more natural. The /n/ literally changes shape to be more like the following consonant. When you use paint, two colors next to each other may blend and create a natural transition. This kind of blending happens between sounds in language, too. Phonological processes like the one just described occur to make them easier to pronounce and seem more natural. When a computer automated voice reads a string of numbers or a sentence aloud, it might sound awkward and choppy because it is pronouncing every sound in isolation. When a human speaks a series of numbers or a sentence aloud, however, that person draws from their phonology layer to make those subtle changes that help them sound more natural. Thus, for language learners to sound more natural and less choppy, we as teachers can help learners understand phonological processes that help them to blend sounds from one to another.

Morphology is the next layer. **Morphology** is the study of word formation, where morphemes, or the smallest unit of language with meaning or function, come together to form words, new and old. Think about a word like *disembarkation*. Although it is one word, it has a lot of parts: first, you have the root word *embark* (verb), then it takes on the prefix *dis-* to change the meaning to the opposite. Then you add the suffix *-ation* to change the part of speech from verb to noun. Roots and affixes, or add-on morphemes, allow us to come up with an infinite number of new words from preexisting words, like *unfriending* or *friendzone*. The morphology layer also tells you that while you can make a word like *unturtlelike* (to be not like a turtle), a word like *disturtlely* breaks the rules somehow. Language learners have to be aware of the word-formation rules of the target language, which not only helps them use and understand existing words and meanings, but also use and understand new ones that come into the vocabulary.

The next layer of the cake is **syntax**, which often turns people off because they think it is either computer language or grammar. A less intimidating way to think about syntax is simply how words come together. There are not a lot of languages that allow you to just put words together however you want and it would still be considered grammatical. Some languages are more permissive than others about word order, but even those have word orders that are more common, or canonical, than others. Syntax is an important layer for language learners because, as many of us know from experience, you cannot just translate a sentence word for word from one language to another. You have to follow the rules of the target language, which can be difficult to learn. In German, for instance, verbs have to go in second position, while in Japanese, the verbs go at the end of a sentence. When you know a language, you know these rules without even realizing you know them, such that when you hear a phrase like *the big red leather cowboy boots*, you know that's right, but there is something odd about *the red cowboy leather big boots*. You might not be able to explain it, but your intuition tells you something has gone awry.

Semantics is the next layer of language. Semantics deals with meaning. Not just the kind of meaning you look up in a dictionary, but really understanding the nuance behind the word, phrase, or sentence. For example, look around you right now and find objects that are *red*. You might find objects that are redder than others, some of which may just barely pass as red. Now, what if you were asked to identify something that is *red-red*. As in, *really* truly red. Suddenly, the field narrows, and you might find yourself excluding some objects because they are too light or too dark or too orangey. *Red-red* isn't an entry you are going to find in a dictionary, nor is the definition consistent from person to person. However, you have a certain intuition about it, and the semantics layer of your language competence tells you that.

Pragmatics is the last layer of language, the layer that deals with how language is used. Pragmatics gives you information about what is appropriate, what is permissible, what makes sense to say given known information, and how you use language to achieve certain acts, like apologizing, thanking, insinuating, or insulting. For instance, pragmatics tells us why the following conversation is perfectly acceptable:

Steve: Hey, Coco, what's up?
Coco: Not too much.

But why this conversation below does not quite work:

Steve: Hey, Coco, what's up?
Coco: Fine, thank you.

And why this conversation is kind of rude or, at least, eye-roll inducing:

Steve: Hey, Coco, what's up?
Coco: The sky.

Pragmatics tends to be more difficult to teach and learn because not only does it utilize the sounds and words and sentences you build from knowledge of the other layers, but you have to understand context and nuance.

These six layers—phonetics, phonology, morphology, syntax, semantics, and pragmatics—exist in all human languages, dialects, and creoles. Every language, however "primitive" it may be considered by society or how frowned-upon it might be by people in power, has a full-fledged system containing all these layers. Signed languages have phonetics and phonology too, as we will later discuss. There is no such thing as a language that simply does not have one of these layers. If you look closely, it will be there.

1.4 Linguistic Competence

Now, let's circle back to the original question: *what do you know when you know a language?* Knowing a language means you need to know all of these components of language. As a learner, you cannot learn just the phonetics layer but ignore the syntax layer. In other words, you might have excellent pronunciation in Arabic, but if you have no idea how to string words together, you cannot really communicate. Similarly, you may know how to string words together in Arabic, but if you don't know what they mean, then it's empty and useless. Or you might have excellent semantic and pragmatic skills, but if your pronunciation is so nontargetlike that people cannot understand you, then you cannot communicate either. When you know a language, you need to have at least some competence in every layer. You do not need to have mastery of every layer to communicate, of course, but you cannot get by without some of each component.

This knowledge of the components is what we call **linguistic competence**. As speakers (or signers) of a language, you have this knowledge of the layers to some extent. Language acquisition, therefore, is the gaining of this linguistic competence. We have mentioned several times as we went over the layers the importance of intuition when analyzing language. Your linguistic competence is what allows you to form your language and also what tells you whether something sounds off or not. However, there is an important distinction between knowledge and awareness. Having the knowledge does not necessarily mean that you are aware of these components and their intricacies. People use very complex linguistic processes all day every day, but most people are not aware of what those processes are or even that they are using them. This is especially true if you learned a language as a child. No one sits down a baby, hands her a notebook, and explains the word order rules of her language. Because language learning tends to happen in natural environments—most often in the home—when you are a baby or small child, you are not aware that you are using the subjunctive mood, labiodental fricative, or nasal assimilation. You just do it because it sounds good and your gut tells you whether something sounds off or not. You know it when you hear it. This is similar to learning to walk. You don't have to know what gravity is or how the human muscular system works in order to walk. You might have excellent competence in forming noun phrases but not know how to describe it or even put a name to it.

This is where teachers who are native speakers of the target language struggle a bit. If you are a native Italian speaker and you are teaching Italian to English-speaking students, it could be somewhat difficult to put yourself into your students' shoes because you don't remember the process of learning to speak Italian: you probably learned it at home with your family as a small child. You did not learn Italian sitting in a classroom like your students. Same goes for many ESL teachers who did not have to learn English in a classroom, but rather at home with their family. You might not have thought about how *few* and *a few* can have quite different meanings: *Few people showed up to the meeting* versus *A few people showed up to the meeting.* However, by studying your language objectively like a linguist, you become aware of the structure and components of the language, making it that much easier and more helpful when you teach it.

It is also important to mention that even if a person is not a fluent speaker of a language—say, an intermediate student of ESL—they still have linguistic competence, and therefore some intuition about the language. As language learners become more and more proficient in the language, they develop more targetlike intuitions that tell them that something sounds right or wrong in the target language. This is important because it gives a lot of credit to the language learner. Your intermediate student might not have the complexity that your advanced students have in their language, but they have some linguistic competence—knowledge about the layers of language—that allows them to then build on it.

1.5 Myths and Truths About Human Language

Before we delve further into the layers of language, it is important for teachers to be aware of the common myths and misconceptions of language. Because language is such a pervasive part of human life, it is easy for these myths and misconceptions to start, spread, and become ingrained in our systems of belief. Next we discuss a few that are especially relevant for language teachers.

Myth 1: Some languages are not as developed as others. Myths like this one stem from people's lack of understanding of the complexity of languages. People usually make this kind of comment regarding languages that are spoken by minority groups or indigenous peoples. The fact is, all languages have all of the layers of languages we discussed, but some of these languages that are less powerful in society are not studied as often, and therefore misunderstood to be less developed. By claiming that a language (or dialect or creole) is not as developed as another language, we fail to recognize the systematic complexities that the language has. It not only belittles the language but it also belittles the people who speak it. As an objective study of language, linguistics shows us that despite social hierarchies amongst languages, every single one has a system of rules governing its sounds, structure, meaning, and use.

Myth 2: We need to preserve language to keep it from changing. You may have heard (or said!) such statements as "young people are ruining the language" or "people don't speak correctly anymore". There tends to be negative reactions to languages changing. However, all languages change over time. What we know as modern-day English is nothing like Old English or Middle English; if you went back in time and found people that speak Middle English, you would not be able to understand them at all. The fact is, all languages change over time. Why? Language is human behavior, and human behavior—as we well know—changes all the time. People sometimes feel threatened by changes in their language and believe that it is our job to maintain that "integrity". Try as we may, language change is a natural process that has been ongoing since the beginning of human language. The only time that a language does not change is when there are no speakers left.

Myth 3: We need to teach students the correct way to speak and write. While there are some varieties of languages that are more accepted by academic and professional communities, there is no such thing as one correct way to speak and write. Even the so-called newscaster dialect varies regionally. In fact, language variation—or different people saying things differently—is as normal as people who have different skin color or different hair types. Of course, it is important to demonstrate to students that there are certain varieties or styles that are more expected for academic purposes, but it is equally important for students to learn that using that same variety and style could ostracize them in social situations. You would not greet a friend the same way you would write an email to your boss's boss. Rather than teaching students the idea of correctness, it is more in their best interest to expose them to a wide variety of the ways that people actually use language.

1.6 Descriptive Linguistics

This brings us to **descriptive linguistics**. We have said before that linguists study languages scientifically and objectively—or essentially, *describe* the language as it is. This is what descriptive linguistics is: a scientific and objective description of language. In contrast, **prescriptive linguistics** tells people what is proper or improper language and how they should use the language—they *prescribe* what people should be doing. Some examples of prescriptive rules you may have heard are as follows:

Don't end a sentence with a preposition.
Use nominative pronouns after the verb *to be*.

Prescriptive grammar rules are like social etiquette rules. They have the tenor of proper rules for society, like *Don't put your elbows on the table* or *Dishes should be passed counterclockwise*. The problem with these prescriptive grammar rules (and maybe etiquette rules as well) is that they do not describe what people actually do. People end sentences with prepositions all the time, and not ending the sentences with a preposition might make you sound overly formal or stilted.

What are you looking for? vs. For what are you looking?
Who'd you talk to? vs. To whom did you talk?

Using nominative pronouns after the verb *to be* makes you sound overly grandiose.

It's me. vs. It is I.

If we encourage our students to follow the prescriptive rules, they will quickly realize that other speakers of the target language do not use it except in the most formal cases. If they use a sentence like *To whom did you talk?* to a friend or knock on the door and announce *It is I*, they will likely fall victim to some light mocking. That is the danger of prescriptive rules and prescriptivism. Instead, by describing the way people actually use language—in informal, neutral, and formal contexts—students are able to learn the complex nature of how their target language functions in real life.

1.7 How to Use This Book

What will this book do for you? At its core, this book is an introduction to linguistics. But unlike many intro books, this one is specifically written and tailored for language teachers, especially ESL, bilingual, world language, and heritage language educators. Because this book is designed for teachers, the lens through which we look at linguistics is through that of language acquisition and teaching. As we delve further into each layer of language, we will highlight areas that are especially pertinent for language learning and teaching, as well as areas that learners might struggle with in each layer.

This book is not a how-to for teaching language. Rather, this book trains language teachers to be linguists themselves. This entails two major skills. The first is to train language teachers to observe language objectively, looking at it "in the wild" as it is used by actual speakers. As we explore the topics of each chapter, the exercises and activities at the end of each chapter may ask you to think of examples from the language(s) you speak and/or teach, and also examples from students learning the target language. Secondly, the book will train you to analyze language. It is quite helpful for teachers to be able to identify patterns in language and use them to help students understand how the language works, as well as identify patterns in the students' errors so teachers can address them and use them to inform their teaching. With these two skills—objective observation and language analysis—the linguist-teacher can really get at the heart of what makes the target language tick, and how to get their students to the next level.

Additionally, this book is not a description of one single language. It considers all languages, and the concepts and skills you learn are meant to serve as a gateway. If you want to study the phonetics of Nahuatl, the syntax of Greek, or the pragmatics of Inuktitut, you will be able to do that. This book will have given you the basic tools to pursue further study into the topics you are interested in. If you get a student in your class who speaks a language you have never heard of (don't be embarrassed, this is very common), you will have the skills to read academic texts and learn more about how that language works. If you are not sure why your French students are having trouble with grammatical gender and want to read about how you can help them, this book will have prepared you to crack that literature.

And if you are a language lover at heart—you love how meaning is created, you love new sounds, you love diagramming sentences—then this book will open your eyes to patterns in the languages you hear all around you that you may have never noticed before. This book can be used as a main text or as a supplementary text in linguistics courses in teacher education programs. At the end of each chapter, **Further Reading** will direct readers to additional resources, and **Exercises** will reinforce the concepts reviewed. In addition, the **Voices From the Classroom** boxes found in every chapter feature first-hand accounts of teachers who have used their knowledge of linguistics to help language learners. The **Glossary** at the end of the book lists key words and phrases, which are bolded the first time they are used in the text.

2 Phonetics
The Sounds of Language

2.1 Introduction

This chapter describes the physiological mechanisms of speech production and how we use articulators in the vocal tract to produce specific sounds. It will explain why a phonetic transcription is necessary to represent sounds in different languages and introduce the International Phonetic Alphabet. We will practice transcribing our own speech using these symbols and learn to group sounds into different classes based on their articulatory and acoustic properties. In addition, we will learn how a focus on prosodic properties (e.g., intonation, stress, and length), in addition to phonetic properties of individual sounds, can facilitate our teaching of pronunciation to second language learners.

In this chapter, we begin with individual sounds, the smallest unit of language. We normally do not think about how sounds are produced in our native languages. The reason that language teachers learn phonetics is to be sensitized to the properties of sounds in different languages—how they are produced (articulatory properties), and what they sound like (acoustic properties)—so that they can help their students to accurately distinguish and produce different sounds. In order to be effective in this endeavor, teachers will want to become familiar with the phonetic inventories of not only English but also the students' native languages so they can identify potential areas of difficulty for the students.

2.2 Why Do We Need a Phonetic Alphabet?

A good phonetic transcription system should have an unambiguous and consistent relationship between written symbols and the sounds that they represent. Each symbol should represent one sound only, and each sound should have only one symbol. The reason that we cannot use the English spelling system to describe sounds is that there is no one-to-one correspondence between English orthography and the sounds it represents. English spelling is highly irregular—the same letter can represent different sounds, or the same sound can be represented by different letters. For example, the letter *s* can represent a number of different sounds in English writing. It can represent the [s] sound in words such as *sun, fast, phonetics*, the [z] sound in *is, use, thieves* or the [ʒ] sound in words like *pleasure, leisure* or no sound at all in *aisle, island, debris*. Conversely, the [i] sound in English can be written using different letters of the English alphabet, as in *see, sea, icy, ceiling, scenic, ravine, brief*. Additionally, the English alphabet is not able to accurately represent sounds that are not in English, such as the [ħ] sound in Arabic or the click sounds in Xhosa.

A phonetic alphabet solves these problems by representing each sound in human speech with a single symbol. Using a phonetic alphabet enables us to transcribe spoken language consistently and accurately. In this book, we will use the International Phonetic Alphabet (IPA), found in the inside back cover of this book (IPA Chart, 2015). The IPA is applicable to all spoken human languages and can be used to describe the sounds of any language. The symbols in the IPA are enclosed in slashes / / or brackets [ ] to indicate that the transcription is phonetic. The IPA does not represent the spelling system of any particular language.

2.3 Articulatory Phonetics: How Sounds Are Produced

Most speech sounds are made by pushing air out of the lungs. Try talking while breathing in and you will notice it's much more difficult than talking while breathing out. Air from the lungs goes up the trachea (also known as the windpipe) and into the larynx, where it passes through the space between the **vocal cords**, called the **glottis**. After the air passes through the glottis, it goes through the tube in the throat called the **pharynx**. Then the air goes out of the **oral cavity** through the mouth, or out of the **nasal cavity** through the nose. Sounds made when the vocal cords are vibrating are called **voiced**, while those made when the vocal cords are apart are called **voiceless**. To hear the difference between a voiced and a voiceless sound, put your fingertips lightly on your throat and say a long *s* sound (like a snake). You should feel no vibration as the vocal cords are separated to make this voiceless sound. Now with your fingertips still on your throat, say a long *z* sound. You will feel a vibration of the vocal cords for this voiced sound.

The difference in voiced and voiceless sounds is important for distinguishing sounds. Table 2.1 lists voiceless consonants in English in the left column and their voiced counterparts in the right column. The underlined sounds in the first row, [p] and [b], differ only in voicing. To check this for yourself, put your fingertips on your throat and say just the underlined consonant in each of these words. Say [p] and [b] alternately—[p, b, p, b, p, b]. Notice that both of these sounds are formed in the same way in the mouth. The only difference is that [p] is voiceless whereas [b] is voiced. The same goes for [f] and [v], for [θ] and [ð], for [s] and [z], and so on.

The air passages above the larynx are called the **vocal tract.** Figure 2.1 shows the principal parts of the vocal tract that can be used to make sounds.

Table 2.1 Voiceless Consonants and Their Voiced Counterparts

Voiceless	Voiced
pad [p]	bad [b]
face [f]	vase [v]
thigh [θ]	thy [ð]
see [s]	zee [z]
dilution [ʃ]	delusion [ʒ]
rich [ʧ]	ridge [ʤ]
tame [t]	dame [d]
coal [k]	goal [g]

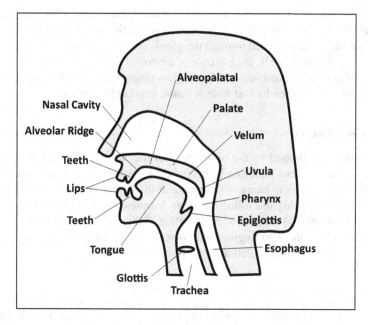

Figure 2.1 The Vocal Tract

These are called **articulators**. The lips and teeth are visible articulators in the front part of the mouth. Just behind the upper teeth is a small protuberance that can be felt with the tip of the tongue, called the **alveolar ridge**. Behind the alveolar ridge is the **hard palate**, a bony structure in the roof of the mouth. Going further back you will find the **soft palate, or velum**. If you have difficulty curling up the tongue far enough to touch the soft palate, you may need to use a fingertip to feel it. The soft palate is a muscular flap that can be raised to press against the back wall of the pharynx to prevent air from escaping through the nose. When this happens, the air can go out only through the mouth, resulting in an **oral sound**. When the soft palate is lowered, however, the air goes out through the nose, resulting in a **nasal sound**. At the lower end of the soft palate is the **uvula**, a fleshy extension that hangs above the throat.

The most important articulator is the **tongue**, a fleshy muscular organ that can produce incredibly fine and complex movements. The tongue can be raised, lowered, pushed forward or pulled back. There are specific names for different parts of the tongue. The **tip** is the narrow area at the front of the tongue. Just behind the tip lies the **blade**. The main mass of the tongue is called the **tongue body**, which may be divided into the **front**, the **center**, and the **back**. The **root** of the tongue lies opposite the back wall of the pharynx.

The sounds of all languages fall into two major categories: consonants and vowels. Consonants are produced with some restriction in the vocal tract as the air from the lungs is pushed through the glottis out of the mouth or the nose. In the production of vowels, the passage of airstream is relatively unobstructed. In the following sections, we will first review characteristics of English consonants and vowels, then look at sounds found in other languages.

2.4 Consonants

Consonants are formed by the *obstruction* of the airstream through the vocal tract. Consonants can therefore be classified according to the place and manner of this obstruction, along with voicing at the larynx. Any given consonant is described by using the following three features: (1) Voicing, (2) Place of Articulation, and (3) Manner of Articulation. Table 2.2 shows the consonants of Mainstream American English, with places of articulation listed from left to right and manners of articulation listed from top to bottom.

Table 2.2 Consonants of Mainstream American English

	Bilabial	Labiodental	Interdental	Alveolar	Post-Alveolar	Palatal	Velar	Glottal
Stop	p b			t d			k g	ʔ
Fricative		f v	θ ð	s z	ʃ ʒ			h
Affricate					ʧ ʤ			
Nasal	m			n			ŋ	
Lateral Liquid				l				
Retroflex Liquid				r				
Glide	ʍ w					j	ʍ w	

Note: Where symbols appear in pairs, the one to the right represents a voiced consonant while the one to the left represents a voiceless consonant.

2.4.1 Places of Articulation

Place of articulation refers to the point where the airstream is obstructed to produce a different sound. Places of articulation are found at the lips, in the oral cavity, in the pharynx, and at the glottis.

(1) **Bilabials** are sounds produced by bringing the two lips together (*bi-* means two, *labial* means lips). In front of a mirror, say words such as *pay, bay, may* and see how the lips come together for the first sound of each of these words. Then say words such as *app, ab, am* and see how the lips come together for the last sound of each word. Then notice what happens as you say the initial sound in words such as *why, win*. This [w] sound involves rounding the lips without stopping the airstream. [ʍ], the voiceless version of [w] occurs in some dialects of English, resulting in different pronunciation of words like *witch* and *which*.

(2) **Labiodentals** are produced by touching the lower lip to the upper front teeth (*labio-* means lips and *dental* means teeth). In front of a mirror, say the words *fine, vine* and see how the lower lip almost touches the upper front teeth for the first sound of each word.

(3) **Interdentals** are produced by inserting the tip of the tongue between the upper and lower teeth. English has two interdental sounds and they are both represented by the *th* in words such as *thigh, thy*.

(4) **Alveolars** are sounds made by raising the front part of the tongue to the alveolar ridge. Say the words *tee, dee, see, zee, knee* and notice how the tongue either touches or almost touches the alveolar ridge for the first part of each word. The [l] is called **lateral** liquid because the tongue is raised to the alveolar ridge with the sides of the tongue down, permitting air to escape laterally over the sides of the tongue. Hold the tongue in position in the last part of the word *tell* while taking in a breath through the mouth. You should feel the incoming air cooling the sides of the tongue. The English [r] is what's called a **retroflex** liquid, produced by curling the tip of the tongue back behind the alveolar ridge.

(5) **Post-Alveolars** (or, sometimes called **alveopalatals**) are produced by raising the front part of the tongue to a point on the hard palate just behind the alveolar ridge. The sound [ʃ] occurs in the beginning of words such as *shy, ship* and its voiced counterpart, [ʒ], occurs in the middle of words such as *measure, pleasure*. [tʃ] and [dʒ], also post-alveolar sounds, occur in the beginning of *cheese* and *geez* respectively.

(6) **Palatals** are produced with the tongue on or near the **palate**, the highest part of the roof of the mouth. The beginning sound in the words *yes, you* is a palatal sound.

(7) **Velars** are sounds made with the tongue on or near the velum, the soft area toward the rear of the roof of the mouth. Velars are the final sounds in words such as *tack, tag, tang*.

(8) **Glottals** are produced by using the **vocal cords** as primary articulators with no other modification of the airstream in the mouth. If the air is stopped at the glottis by tightly closed vocal cords, the sound is called a glottal stop, or [ʔ]. This sound occurs in the exclamation *uh-oh!*, or is used in place of the [t] sound in words such as *kitten, mutton*. The beginning sound in words such as *hi, hen, here* is also a glottal, but air passes through the open glottis.

2.4.2 Manners of Articulation

Manner of articulation refers to the way the airstream is modified by the vocal tract to produce sounds. The lips, tongue, velum, and glottis can be positioned in different ways to produce different sounds.

(1) **Stops** are made when there is a complete closure of the articulators so that air is stopped. There are two possible types of stops. If the air is stopped in the oral cavity but the velum is lowered so that air escapes through the nose, the sound produced is a **nasal stop**. In contrast, if the velum is not lowered, the air cannot escape through the nose, resulting in an **oral stop**. To see how nasal stops are different from oral stops, hold your nose while saying *my nanny*. It will sound something like *bye daddy*. This is because [m] and [b] are produced in the same way by stopping the airflow at the lips. The only difference is that for [m], the velum is lowered to allow the air to go out the nose. Holding your nose while saying [m] prevents the air from escaping through the nose, making it sound more like its oral counterpart, [b]. The same can be said for [n] and [d], which are produced in exactly the same way by having the front part of the tongue touch the alveolar ridge. Holding your nose while saying [n] prevents air from escaping through the nose and makes this nasal stop sound more like its oral counterpart, [d]. The same principle applies to [ŋ] and [g]. Although both the nasal stop and the oral stop can be classified as stops, the term **stop** by itself is typically used to indicate an oral stop, while the term **nasal** is used to indicate a nasal stop.

(2) **Fricatives** are produced when the airstream is partially obstructed to allow air to continuously flow through the mouth. When fricatives are produced, the air passes through a very narrow opening either at the glottis or in the vocal tract, resulting in a continuous turbulent noise, or frication. The beginning consonants in *face, vase, thigh, thy, sue, zoo,* and *ship*, as well as the consonants in the middle of the words *measure* and *aha*, are examples of fricative sounds.

(3) **Affricates** are a combination of two manners of articulation: a stop and a fricative. They are made by a stop closure followed immediately by a slight release of the articulators so that turbulent noise is produced. The beginning consonants in *chewed* and *Jude* are examples of the two affricates in English.

(4) **Nasals** are produced by lowering the velum and opening the nasal passage to the vocal tract. As explained earlier, nasals are sometimes called nasal stops because, just like the oral stops, there is complete obstruction of the airstream in the oral cavity. The only difference between nasal and oral stops is that for nasal stops, the velum is lowered to allow the air to escape through the nasal cavity. English has nasals in three different places of articulation: bilabial, alveolar, and velar.

(5) **Liquids** are consonants that involve substantial constriction of the vocal tract but the constriction is not sufficiently narrow to block the vocal tract or cause friction. There are mainly two types of liquids in English, namely, [l] and [r]. For the lateral liquid [l], the center of the vocal tract is completely obstructed, as in a stop, but air escapes through the sides of the tongue. Try saying the word *hill* and pause your tongue at the [l], then inhale sharply. The sides of your tongue should feel cool with the incoming air. Liquids are typically voiced in English. However, liquids become voiceless after voiceless stops, as in the English words *plead* [pl̥id] and *clay* [kl̥ɛj]. The voiceless lateral is written with an additional phonetic symbol, called a **diacritic**. In this case, the diacritic is a small circle beneath the [l] and denotes voicelessness on a sound that is otherwise voiced.

The other liquid in English is [r]. This sound is made either by curling the tongue tip back into the mouth or by bunching the tongue upward and back in the mouth. This r, which is known as retroflex r, is heard in words such as *rate* and *far* in American English. In IPA, the symbol [r] is reserved for a trilled r, as in Spanish *perro* "dog". The IPA transcribes the retroflex r as [ɹ], but in this book, we will use the symbol [r] for the retroflex r. In some languages, the r is produced by a single tap or a flap of the tongue against the alveolar ridge. In IPA, the flap is transcribed as [ɾ]. In Spanish both the trilled and tapped r occur as in *perro* "dog" and *pero* "but". Some speakers of British English pronounce the r in the word *very* with [ɾ]. Most American English speakers use [ɾ] instead of a [t] or [d] in words like *little* [lɪɾl], and *ladder* [læɾər].

(6) **Glides** are sounds that are made with little or no obstruction of the airstream in the mouth. [w] is made by both rounding the lips and simultaneously raising the back of the tongue toward the velum. For that reason, [w] is called a labio-velar glide. [w̥] is made just like [w], except that it is voiceless. Some English speakers use this sound to distinguish the pronunciation of the word *which* [w̥ɪʧ] from that of *witch* [wɪʧ]. [j] is a palatal glide, which is made by raising the blade of the tongue toward the hard palate as if producing the vowel sound [i]. When occurring in a word, glides must always be either preceded or followed by a vowel. In articulating [w] or [j], the tongue rapidly glides toward or away from a neighboring vowel, hence the term **glide**. For example, in producing *yes* [yɛs], the tongue moves rapidly from the [j] to the [ɛ] vowel. Glides are transition sounds that are sometimes called **semivowels**.

2.5 Consonants in Other Languages

So far we have reviewed consonants in English. In this section, we will consider consonants that are in other languages. Learning to accurately produce these non-English sounds can be challenging but with practice one can achieve reasonable approximations of native pronunciations.

When we examine the IPA consonant chart (found at the top of the inside back cover of this book), we notice that there are three places of articulation that we have not considered so far: the retroflex, uvular, and pharyngeal sounds. Retroflex sounds do not occur in most varieties of English except for those spoken in India. They are produced by curling the tip of the tongue back behind the alveolar ridge. Thus the voiceless retroflex fricative [ʂ] is produced by sliding the tongue back and curling up the tip while saying [s]. You will notice that [ʂ] sounds something like [ʃ]. Similarly, the retroflex stops [ʈ] and [ɖ] are made by curling up the tongue tip while producing [t] and [d]. The curling of the tongue tip gives retroflex sounds an r-like quality.

Uvular sounds are made by raising the back of the tongue toward the uvula. The voiced uvular fricative [ʁ] is used in French words such as *roi* [ʁwa] "king" and *rapide* [ʁapid] "fast". The voiceless uvular fricative [χ] occurs in French after voiceless stops, as in *mètre* [mɛtχ] "meter". The voiceless uvular stop [q] is pronounced like [k], except that the tongue makes contact with the uvula. It occurs in the word [qɑzɑq] "Kazakh" in the Kazakh language. Uvular stops [q] and [ɢ] and uvular nasal [ɴ] occur in some of the indigenous languages of the Americas such as Inuktitut and Quechua.

For most English speakers, pharyngeal sounds are fairly difficult to make. The IPA lists two fricatives in the pharyngeal region, [ħ] and [ʕ], which occur in Semitic languages such as Arabic and Hebrew. Pharyngeal fricatives are made by pulling the tongue root toward the back wall of the pharynx. They occur in words like [ħadiqa] "garden" and [muħammad] "Mohamed" and [ʕarab] "Arab" in Arabic.

Other than uvular and pharyngeal sounds, the majority of non-English sounds that are found in other languages involve different manners of articulation at the same places of articulation as in English. For example, English has bilabial stops and nasals, but no bilabial fricatives. Acoustically, the voiceless and voiced bilabial fricatives, [ɸ] and [β], sound like labiodental fricatives, [f] and [v], but they are made by bringing the lips almost together so that there is a narrow opening between them. In the West African language, Ewe, the use of bilabial or labiodental fricatives results in meaning differences in word pairs such as [èβɛ̀] "Ewe" (the name of the language) and [èvɛ̀] "two". Similarly, Ewe contrasts [ɸ] with [f] in [éɸá] "he polished" and [éfá] "he was cold".

The voiceless palatal fricative [ç] occurs in German in words such as [ɪç] "I" and [nɪçt] "not" and is acoustically similar to the first part of the English word [hju] "hue". The voiceless velar fricative [x], as in the German words [axt] "eight" and [naxt] "night", is made by building up pressure behind the velar closure without completely stopping the airflow as one would when producing

[k]. Spanish has velar fricatives [x] and [ɣ] in words such as [xaβon] "soap" and [xuɣar] "to play".

Voices From the Classroom 2.1—How Knowledge of Students' Native Languages Can Help in Teaching Them English Pronunciation

I noticed that many of my Arabic-speaking ESL students had difficulty pronouncing [ʒ] as in the word *pleasure* [plɛʒər]. But once I realized that Arabic has this sound in words like *Jordan* which is pronounced [ʒordan], I was able to point out to the students that the *s* in *pleasure* is the same sound as the beginning sound in *Jordan*.

Chris McKinnon, Adult ESL Instructor

2.6 Vowels

When we produce vowel sounds, none of the articulators come very close together, and the passage of the airstream is relatively unobstructed. Any given vowel is described by using the following four features: (1) the height of the tongue; (2) the front-back position of the tongue; (3) the degree of lip rounding; and (4) tense-lax gesture of the tongue.

To get a feel for differences in tongue height, place a lollipop on your tongue and say the following words with front vowels: *eat, ate, at*. You will notice that it is not very easy to say *eat* with the lollipop in your mouth, because the lollipop gets in the way of the tongue trying to bunch up toward the roof of the mouth. But as you produce the mid vowel in the word *ate*, the tongue is not as bunched up high in the mouth, leaving more room for the lollipop. It becomes easier still to produce the low vowel in the word *at* because the tongue is completely lowered.

You can try the same thing for the back vowels. With the lollipop on your tongue, say the following words: *ooze, o's, ah's*. You will notice that it is not difficult to say these words with the lollipop in your mouth because all of these vowels require the back of the tongue to move up and down in the mouth. Since the lollipop sits on the front part of the tongue, it does not interfere in the production of the back vowels. Even so, you should feel that it gets progressively easier to say the words as the tongue is progressively lowered.

Figure 2.2 shows the position of the tongue in the words *beet, bait, bet, bat, bot, bought, boat, boot*. In the first four vowels /i, e, ɛ, æ/, the highest point of the tongue is in the front of the mouth. Therefore, these vowels are called **front**

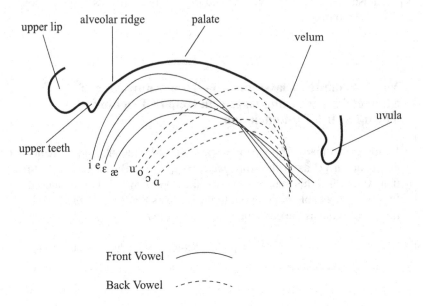

Figure 2.2 Front Vowel ———

Back Vowel -- -- -- --

Figure 2.2 The Positions of the Tongue for the Vowels in "Beet, Bait, Bet, Bat, Bot, Bought, Boat, Boot"

vowels. The tongue is highest in the mouth for the vowel in *beet*, slightly lower for the vowel in *bait*, and lower still for the vowels in *bet* and *bat*. The vowel in *beet* is called a **high** front vowel, while the vowel in bat is called a **low** front vowel. The height of the tongue for the vowels in *bait* and *bet* is between these two extremes, and they are called **mid** front vowels. In the four **back** vowels /ɑ, ɔ, o, u/, the tongue is close to the back surface of the vocal tract. The tongue is highest in the vowel in *boot* and lowest in the vowel in *bot*. Thus the vowel in *boot* is called a high back vowel, while the vowel in *bot* is called a low back vowel. The vowels in *boat* and *bought* are classified as mid back vowels. In addition to the front and back vowels, English has a mid central vowel, which is written with the symbol [ə] to denote the vowel in the first syllable of *about* [əbawt], or with the symbol [ʌ] to denote the vowel in *but* [bʌt]. [ə] and [ʌ] are essentially the same vowel except that [ə] is used to denote a mid central vowel in unstressed syllables while [ʌ] is reserved for stressed (or only) syllables.

Figure 2.3 shows the vowels in English. Notice that the tongue positions in Figure 2.2 roughly correspond to the placement of the symbols in the vowel chart in Figure 2.3. Although the vowel space is neatly divided into high, mid, and low for tongue height, and front, central, and back for placement of the tongue in the front or back of the mouth, it is important to note that there are really no distinct boundaries between one type of vowel and another. Vowels are much more fluid and continuous than consonants. See this for yourself by saying [i] as in *he* and move slowly to [æ] as in *had*. You will notice that you pass through sounds similar to [ɛ] in *head* and [e] in *hey*. It is perfectly possible

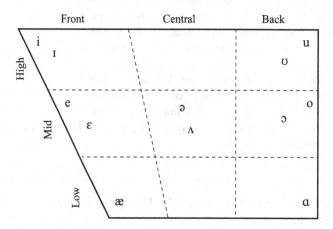

Figure 2.3 The Vowels in English

to make a vowel that is halfway between a mid vowel and a low vowel. In fact, it is possible to make a vowel at any spot on the vowel chart by making ever so slight changes in the shape and placement of the tongue and rounding of the lips. Consonants, on the other hand, are much more distinct from one another. Consider two different manners of articulation—a fricative and a liquid. A sound may be a fricative or a liquid, but it cannot be halfway between the two.

In addition to the height and front-back position of the tongue, vowel quality also depends on the shape of the lips. Look at your lips in a mirror while you say just the vowels in the words *boot, put, boat, bought.* You will notice that your lips are **rounded**. Now say the remaining vowels in the vowel chart in Figure 2.3 while looking in a mirror. You will notice that your lips are **unrounded**.

Finally, the vowels in English can be grouped into **tense** and **lax** vowels. Tense vowels generally require more extreme tongue gesture to reach the outer edges of the vowel space than lax vowels. There are four tense/lax vowel pairs that make a meaning difference in English words: (1) the [i, ɪ] pair as in *beet* and *bit*; (2) the [e, ɛ] pair as in *bait* and *bet;* (3) [u, ʊ] pair as in *boot* and *put*; and (4) the [o, ɔ] pair as in *boat* and *bought.* The difference between the vowels in *bait* and *bet* is that the vowel in *bet* is shorter, lower, and slightly more centralized than the vowel in *bait.* We call the vowel in *bet* a mid front lax vowel, and the vowel in *bait* a mid front tense vowel. Likewise, the lax vowels [ɪ] and [ʊ] are shorter, lower, and slightly more centralized than their tense counterparts [i] and [u].

In summary, the vowels in English can be described using the four aforementioned factors as follows:

[i], as in *beet,* is a high, front, unrounded, tense vowel.
[ɪ], as in *bit,* is a high, front, unrounded, lax vowel.

[e], as in *bait*, is a mid, front, unrounded, tense vowel.

[ɛ], as in *bet*, is a mid, front, unrounded, lax vowel.

[æ], as in *bat*, is a low, front, unrounded, lax vowel.

[u], as in *boot*, is a high, back, rounded, tense vowel.

[ʊ], as in *put*, is a high, back, rounded, lax vowel.

[o], as in *boat*, is a mid, back, rounded, tense vowel.

[ɔ], as in *bought*, is a mid, back, rounded, lax vowel.

[ɑ], as in *bot*, is a low, back, unrounded, lax vowel.

[ə], as in the first syllable of *about*, and [ʌ], as in *but*, is a mid, central, unrounded, lax vowel.

Voices From the Classroom 2.2—Using the Color Vowel Chart

Many of my students have had problems with various vowel sounds in English. Teaching the phonetic symbols was more time consuming than helpful for my students. Now, I use the Color Vowel Chart (https://americanenglish.state.gov/resources/color-vowel-chart) in class to help students remember the vowel sounds. The chart assigns a color and a common object to a vowel sound and helps students recognize the many vowel sounds in English as well as the multitude of vowel sounds for one letter. For instance, if students are challenged by the pronunciation of the word *refugee* (a common mispronunciation in my experience), students would remember *red dress, blue moon*, and *green tea*. These help young students to learn the correct pronunciation of a new word.

Morgan Nixon, ESL Teacher

2.6.1 Diphthongs

Diphthongs can be described as movements from one vowel to another. The first part of the diphthong is usually more prominent than the second, which is often transitory. The tense vowels in American English, [i], [e], [u], and [o], are phonetically diphthongs. This is why in some transcription systems, these vowels are transcribed as [ij], [ej], [uw], and [ow] respectively. Most other languages use "pure" vowels instead of diphthongs for these sounds. As such, English speakers should learn to hear the glides in these tense vowels and avoid them as they learn to speak other languages, unless they are specifically called for. For example, many American English speakers typically pronounce the Spanish word *peso* as /pejsow/. But if the goal is to sound more like a native Spanish speaker, one should use pure vowels and say /peso/. In addition to [ij], [ej], [uw], and [ow], English has other diphthongs such as [aw], as in *brow*, [ɔj], as in *boy*, [aj], as in *buy*.

2.6.2 Phonics vs. Phonetics—What's the Difference?

At this point, it may be helpful to consider a question often asked by language arts teachers, namely, "what is the difference between phonics and phonetics?" Phonics is a teaching tool used to help children who already speak English to learn to read in English. As explained earlier, English orthography has a highly irregular spelling. While variability in spelling is found in both consonants and vowels, there is far greater variability when it comes to writing vowel sounds than consonant sounds. For example, the [o] sound can be written in at least six different ways (oval, nose, boat, bow, toe, though). Then there are words containing the letter o that sound like [ɑ] in American English (box, mop, hot, frog). For children who are just beginning to read, the label "short o" is helpful in associating the [ɑ] sound in words like box, mop, hot, and frog with the letter o written on the page.

Thus, by grouping vowels into "long" and "short" categories, phonics helps children recognize letter patterns in written text. As can be seen in Table 2.3, for each of the five vowels, a, e, i, o, and u, there is a long version and a short version (long e, short e, long a, short a, and so on). Notice that the words *beet* and *bet* which have the "long e" and "short e" sounds respectively, have e's in them. Similarly, *bait* and *bat* which have the "long a" and "short a" sounds respectively, have a's in them. The "long" and "short" characterizations roughly correspond to tense and lax vowels respectively. Thus, "long e", or the sound transcribed in IPA as [i], is a tense vowel while "short e", transcribed in IPA as [ɛ], is a lax vowel.

One may ask, "if the sound [i] corresponds to the long *e* sound, why is it represented with the letter *i*?" This is because in most languages that use the

Table 2.3 Phonics vs. Phonetics

What the vowel is called in phonics	Words in English with the vowel	How the vowel is transcribed using phonetic symbols
long e	beet	[i]
short e	bet	[ɛ]
long a	bait	[e]
short a	bat	[æ]
long i	bite	[aj]
short i	bit	[ɪ]
long o	boat	[o]
short o	bot	[ɑ]
long u	butte	[ju]
short u	but	[ʌ]

Roman alphabet, the long *e* sound is written with the letter *i*. For example, in Spanish, the letter *i* in words such as *picante* ("spicy") and *dinero* ("money") are pronounced with the long *e* or [i] sound. Similarly, the letter *i* in words such as *midi* ("noon") and *piscine* ("swimming pool") in French are pronounced with the long *e* or [i] sound.

A phonetic transcription, on the other hand, is a more accurate description of individual sounds, with each phonetic symbol representing only one sound. Additionally, when we look at the phonetic chart, it provides information about how and where to produce the sound. In order for teachers to correctly identify pronunciation difficulties of ESL students, they need to have an accurate and reliable way to refer to individual sounds. For students who are learning English for the first time as adolescents or adults, the "long" and "short" vowel characterizations will not make much sense since they do not already know how to speak English.

2.7 Vowels in Other Languages

Compared to many of the world's languages, English has a relatively large vowel inventory with eleven monophthongs in stressed syllables (check out Vowel Quality Inventories in the World Atlas of Language Structures Online at: http://wals.info/chapter/2). The five-vowel system of Spanish is much more common among the world's languages. Hundreds of languages have only five or six contrasting vowels (Japanese, Mandarin, and Swahili). It should be noted, however, a given symbol on these charts does not have the same value for all the languages. As we reviewed earlier in this chapter, tense vowels in English behave more like diphthongs. In contrast, the five vowels in Spanish are more pure vowels. Figure 2.4 shows the vowel inventories of English, Spanish, and French.

French has three front rounded vowels [y, ø, œ]. The high front rounded vowel [y] is produced by saying [i] with the lips rounded. To make this sound, begin by making the [i] sound, then slowly bring your lips to a rounded position while keeping the tongue position for [i]. The [y] sound is used in French words such as *tu* [ty] ("you" informal) and *vu* [vy] ("saw"), and contrasts with the high back vowel [u] in *tous* [tu] ("all") and *vous* [vu] ("you" formal). Similarly, the mid front rounded vowel [ø] is produced with a tongue position as in [e], but with rounded lips.

Earlier in this chapter, we saw that English has two kinds of stops: oral stops [p, b, t, d, k, g] and nasal stops [m, n, ŋ]. Vowels, on the other hand, are most often oral sounds. But vowels may be nasalized if the velum is lowered to allow part of the airstream to flow through the nose. Nasalization commonly occurs in vowels next to nasal consonants (more on this in the next chapter), but it can be a contrastive property in some languages like French, Hindi, and Navajo. In French, for instance, using an oral or a nasal vowel results in different words, as in *mais* [mɛ] ("but") and *main* [mɛ̃] ("hand"), and *beau* [bo] ("beautiful") and *bon* [bõ] ("good"). The diacritic [˜] placed

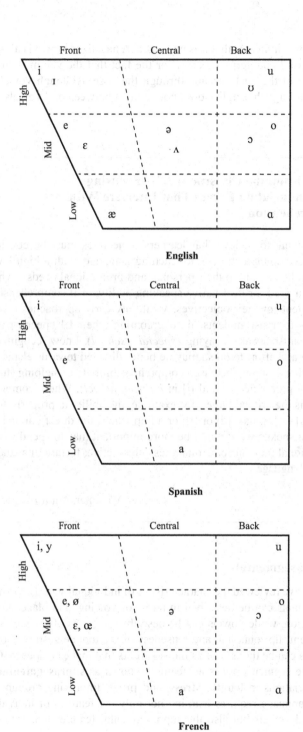

Figure 2.4 Vowels in English, Spanish, and French

above a vowel indicates that it is nasalized. A nasalized vowel is almost identical to its oral counterpart except for the fact that the velum is lowered to allow some of the air to escape through the nose. Although vowels can be nasalized in English, English does not contrast between oral vowels and their nasal counterparts.

Voices From the Classroom 2.3—Focusing on Pronunciation Errors That Interfere With Comprehension

I have come to believe that learners' objectives must be considered when developing a strategy to teaching language, with a high level of attention being paid to their personal and professional needs—whether there is a need for near-native speaking ability, or if comprehensibility is sufficient for their objectives. While my early approaches involved attempts to assist students in "overcoming" their L1 speech patterns (e.g., Spanish speakers saying *especial, eschool*), I now recognize that the time and effort to do so may be better directed towards elements of speech that promote increased comprehensibility (e.g., helping students correctly pronounce [ɪ] and [i] in *bit/beet, fit/feet*). Where comprehensibility is the critical target, for example, the ability to properly form a plural [s] or [z]; past [d] or [t]; or a flap versus the direct phonetic version of a spoken word might be more important than to spend valuable instructional time on some other, less obstructive, feature of a student's spoken language.

Steven Wagoner, Adult ESL Teacher

2.8 Suprasegmentals

So far we have reviewed the characteristics of individual sounds. We have seen that consonants can be described in terms of voicing, and place and manner of articulation, while vowels can be described in terms of tongue height and advancement, lip rounding, and tenseness of the tongue gesture. Consonants and vowels can be thought of as the **segments** that make up speech. Over and above these segments are other features known as **suprasegmentals**. These include variations in **length**, **stress**, and **pitch**. Improving pronunciation in a second language requires learning not only the features of individual consonants and vowels but also the suprasegmental features that extend across multiple segments in an utterance.

2.8.1 Length

The first suprasegmental feature we will consider is **length**. In many languages, differences in the duration of segments can be meaningful. For example, Japanese contrasts between short and long vowels in words like [ojisan] "uncle" and [oji:san] "grandfather", as well as [obasan] "aunt" and [oba:san] "grandmother". The colon [:] placed after a vowel indicates that it is lengthened. In Thai, vowel duration is linked to differences in meaning in words such as [tak] "to dip up" versus [ta:k] "to dry", and [khut] "to dig" versus [khu:t] "to scrape". Some languages contrast short and long consonants. In Arabic, consonant lengthening results in meaning difference in [qabala] "he accepted" versus [qabbala] "he kissed". In Finnish, [kuka] means "who" while [kukka] means "flower". The doubled consonant in these examples reflects lengthening.

2.8.2 Stress

Consonants and vowels together form syllables, which make up utterances. In any utterance, some syllables are perceived to be more prominent than others and are said to have greater **stress**. Stressed syllables are generally longer, louder, and higher in pitch than unstressed syllables. In English, stress can have a grammatical function. For example, variations in stress are used to distinguish between a noun and a verb in English. When you say the words *(an) ínsert* versus *(to) insért, (a) cóntrast* versus *(to) contrást*, or *(a) présent* versus *(to) presént*, you will notice that the stress is on the first syllable in the nouns whereas it is on the last syllable in the verbs. Stress can also be used to emphasize certain words in expressions like *She's wearing a pínk dress (not a blue dress)*, as opposed to *She's wearing a pink dréss (not a suit)*.

English uses several levels of stress in multisyllabic words such as *démocràt, demócracỳ, dèmocrátic, dèmocrátically*. An acute accent ['] placed over the vowel marks the most prominent or **primary stress** whereas a grave accent ['] marks the second most prominent or **secondary stress**. In IPA, ['] is placed before the beginning of a syllable with primary stress, while [ˌ] is placed before the syllable with secondary stress. Thus, the same words would be transcribed as ['dɛməˌkræt], [dəˈmɑkrəˌsi], [ˌdɛməˈkrærɪk], [ˌdɛməˈkrærɪkli].

Placement of stress is predictable and relatively straightforward in some languages. In French, for example, stress is placed on the final syllable of a word. In Spanish, stress is placed on the penultimate (second to last) syllable in words that end in a vowel or *n* or *s* (e.g., *náda, ésta, éstas, cántan*) and on the final syllable in words that end in a consonant other than *n* or *s* (e.g., *hablár, libertád, comér*). However, placement of stress varies according to the word in English, which poses significant problems for those trying to learn it as a second language. Although there are some rules, they are rather complicated and unwieldy. Nonetheless there are some useful ways to teach English stress patterns to second language learners (see Voices from the Classroom 2.4— Teaching English Stress Patterns).

Voices From the Classroom 2.4—Teaching English Stress Patterns

- Raise awareness and build confidence

    Some learners love to learn about the "technical" side of language, while others like to "feel" or "see" the language more, hearing the music of word stress or seeing the shapes of the words. Try to use a variety of approaches: helping students to engage with English in different ways will help them in their goal to become more proficient users of the language.

- Mark the stress

    Use a clear easy-to-see way of marking stress on the board and on handouts for students.

- Integrate word stress into your lessons

    You don't need to teach separate lessons on word stress. Instead, you can integrate it into your normal lessons. The ideal time to focus students' attention on it is when introducing vocabulary. Quickly and simply elicit the stress pattern of the word from the students (as you would the meaning) and mark it on the board. Drill it, too!

- Troubleshooting

    Initially, many students (and teachers!) find it difficult to hear word stress. A useful strategy is to focus on one word putting the stress on its different syllables in turn. For example: com**pu**ter **com**puter

- Say the word in the different ways for the students, really exaggerating the stressed syllable and compressing the unstressed ones. Ask the students which version of the word sounds "the best" or "the most natural." By hearing the word stressed incorrectly, students can more easily pick out the correct version.

Excerpted from a web article written by Emma Pathare, Teacher, Trainer, Dubai (Retrieved June 8, 2016 from: www.teachingenglish.org.uk/article/word-stress)

2.8.3 Pitch

Pitch is the auditory property of a sound that can be placed on a scale that ranges from low to high. It correlates to fundamental frequency and depends on the rate of vibration of the vocal folds. We can vary pitch by controlling the tension of the vocal folds and the amount of air that passes through the glottis.

While more tense vocal folds and greater air pressure lead to higher pitch, less tense vocal folds and lower air pressure result in lower pitch. There are mainly two types of controlled pitch movement that are found in the world's languages: (1) **tone** and (2) **intonation**.

Pitch differences that change the meaning of a word are called **tones**. Languages that exploit this feature are called **tonal languages**. They include many of the languages spoken in Southeast Asia (e.g., Burmese, Thai, Vietnamese), all varieties of Chinese, African languages such as Zulu, Luganda, and Igbo, as well as many of the Native languages of the Americas (e.g., Navajo, Cherokee, Zuni). For example, in Mandarin Chinese four different tones can combine with the syllable *ma* to produce different words: (1) *mā* (high level) "mother"; (2) *má* (high rising) "hemp"; (3) *mǎ* (low falling rising) "horse"; (4) *mà* (high falling) "scold". Similarly, Thai has five tones that result in differences in meaning: (1) /kʰāː/ (mid) "stick"; (2) /kʰàː/ (low) "galangal—an Asian plant of the ginger family"; (3) /kʰâː/ (falling) "value"; (4) /kʰáː/ (high) "to trade"; (5) /kʰǎː/ (rising) "leg".

Both Mandarin Chinese and Thai have **contour tones**, which can be described in terms of shifts in pitch rather than single points within a pitch range. The falling and rising tones in the preceding Mandarin Chinese and Thai examples illustrate contour tones. In contrast, **register tones** are level tones that describe specific points within a pitch range. The distinguishing feature in languages with register tones is the relative difference between the pitches such as high, mid, or low, not the shape of their movements. Luganda, Zulu, and Hausa are examples of register tone languages with two tones—high and low. Yoruba is an example of a tonal language with three tones—high, mid, and low. In a tonal language, it is not the absolute pitch of the syllables that is important but the relative pitch among different syllables. A tone is perceived as high if it is high relative to other pitches around it produced by the same speaker.

Intonation refers to pitch movement that is not related to differences in word meaning. Thus, in a **non-tonal language** such as English, whether one pronounces the word *sandwich* with a rising pitch or a falling pitch makes no difference to the meaning of the word. But intonation can be used to convey broader linguistic meaning in both tonal and non-tonal languages. For example, the falling pitch we hear at the end of a statement in English such as *He had a sandwich* signals that the utterance is complete. But a rising pitch at the end of the same utterance would signal that the speaker is asking a question (*He had a sandwich?*). If the word *sandwich* were part of a list, it would be pronounced with an intonation that first falls and then rises again slightly. Thus in the statement *He had a sandwich, a bag of chips, and a large soda* the words *sandwich* and *chips* would be marked by a rising intonation to indicate that the speaker is not finished speaking while the sentence-final word *soda* is pronounced with a falling intonation.

2.9 Syllable-Timed vs. Stress-Timed Languages

The world's languages can be classified into two main categories: **syllable-timed** and **stress-timed**. In syllable-timed languages, the more syllables there are, the more time it takes to say something because each syllable is approximately the same length as other syllables. Examples of syllable-timed languages include Spanish, French, Korean, and Japanese. English is a stress-timed language, where syllables are not similar in length. A stress-timed language is a language where the stressed syllables are said at approximately regular intervals, and unstressed syllables shorten to fit this rhythm. Oral speech in English is rhythmic and moves from one stressed syllable to the next stressed syllable. Everything in between is shortened to fit the rhythm set by stressed syllables. To see how this works, use a metronome (you can access a free metronome online from sites such as www.metronomeonline.com/). Set the metronome to a comfortable walking tempo (around 80 to 90 beats per minute) and read the following sentences one by one, making sure that each stressed syllable falls *on* the beat and unstressed syllables fall *in between* the beats. Notice that, as more and more syllables are added, it still takes the same amount of time to produce each sentence. Each sentence is said in exactly three beats, which correspond to the number of stressed syllables in each sentence.

Kíds pláy gámes. (3 syllables)
The kíds pláy gámes. (4 syllables)
The kíds pláy the gámes. (5 syllables)
The kíds will pláy the gámes. (6 syllables)
The kíds will be pláying the gámes. (7 syllables)

If English were a syllable-timed language, it would take more time to produce the longer sentences. English learners whose native language is a syllable-timed language have a tendency to assign equal length to each syllable in English, whether stressed or not. These learners would do well to distinguish between stressed and unstressed syllables and learn to reduce the vowels in unstressed syllables. The reverse is true for English speakers who are learning a syllable-timed language like Spanish and French. English speakers may set the metronome to the syllable level and learn to pronounce each syllable with full vowels.

2.10 The Importance of the [ə] in Improving Pronunciation in English

When words in English are produced in isolation, at least one syllable is stressed. In case of words that are composed of one syllable, that syllable will be stressed. Thus, each of the words in the sentence *She said that to you and me*, when produced in isolation, would sound something like this:

[ʃi], [sɛd], [ðæt], [tu], [ju], [ænd], [mi]

However, when the words are said in quick succession in conversation, they undergo considerable change. Some words will be completely unstressed, the vowel may be reduced to [ə] or may disappear altogether, and one or more of the consonants may be dropped or altered. Thus, *She said that to you and me* in connected speech might sound like: [ʃɪ 'sɛd ðət tə 'ju ən 'mi]. Notice that the vowels in unstressed words are reduced and the final consonant in the word "and" is dropped.

The mid central vowel in English, [ə] (also known as *schwa*), is critical in English because vowels in unstressed syllables are often reduced to it. Let's see how placement of stress changes vowel quality. Consider the words *emphátic* [ɛm'fæʃɪk] and *émphasis* ['ɛmfəsɪs]. Both have three syllables. However, notice that the stress falls on the second syllable in *emphatic* whereas it falls on the first syllable in *emphasis*. The low front vowel [æ] is reduced to a mid central vowel [ə] in an unstressed vowel. Teachers sometimes hear English learners pronounce the second vowel in *emphasis* as [æ]. To help these students, teachers might point out that the stress falls on the first syllable in *emphasis* and that the vowel in the unstressed second syllable is reduced to a [ə].

To help students achieve more natural-sounding and less stilted pronunciation in English, teachers can review the different ways that some of the monosyllabic function words in English are pronounced in stressed or unstressed positions (see Table 2.4).

Since English is a stress-timed language, English speakers tend to pronounce full vowels only when they are in stressed syllables. The remaining syllables are reduced, usually to [ə]. However, English speakers learning other languages will want to produce each vowel as a full vowel when speaking other languages.

Table 2.4 How Functions Words Are Pronounced Differently in Stressed vs. Unstressed Positions

Function Word	Stressed	Unstressed	Example in Conversation
and	ænd	ənd, ən, nd, n̩	'Tom and 'Jerry ['tam n̩ 'dʒeri]
as	æz	əz	as 'fast as light [əz 'fæst əz lait]
at	æt	ət	'see you at 'noon ['si ju ət 'nun]
can	kæn	kən	I can 'dig. [aɪ kən 'dɪg]
has	hæz	həz, əz	'He has done it. ['hi əz dən ɪt]
he	hi	hɪ, ɪ	Will he 'look? [wɪl ɪ 'lʊk]
to	tu	tə	You 'have to 'tell her. [ju 'hæv tə 'tɛl ər]

Recommended Websites

Interactive IPA Chart with Audio Recordings
https://www.internationalphoneticassociation.org/IPAcharts/inter_
    chart_2018/IPA_2018.html
The World Atlas of Language Structures Online
http://wals.info/
Type IPA Phonetic Symbols
https://ipa.typeit.org/

Further Reading

Ashby, P. (2011). *Understanding phonetics*. Oxon, UK: Hodder Education.
Collins, B., & Mees, I. M. (2013). *Practical phonetics and phonology: A resource book for students* (3rd ed.). London and New York: Routledge.
Ladefoged, P., & Johnson, K. (2015). *A course in phonetics* (7th ed.). Stamford, CT: Cengage Learning.

Exercises

1. Using the words from the Word Bank, fill in the names of the vocal organs
    in Figure 2.5.

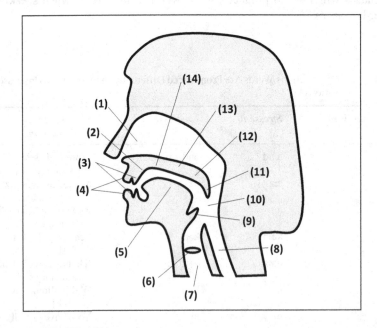

Figure 2.5 The Vocal Tract

> **Word Bank**
> nasal cavity, uvula, teeth, lips, velum (soft palate), palate, tongue, glottis,
> alveolar ridge, esophagus, epiglottis, alveopalatal, pharynx, trachea

2. Following the examples below, provide three-part description of each consonant, starting with voicing, place of articulation, and manner of articulation in that order.

   a) /p/—voiceless bilabial stop
   b) /g/—voiced velar stop
   c) /f/—voiceless labiodental fricative
   d) /s/—
   e) /n/—
   f) /l/—
   g) /θ/—
   h) /ʤ/—

3. Transcribe the following words:

   a) image [   ]
   b) choice [   ]
   c) grief [   ]
   d) advise [   ]
   e) advice [   ]
   f) remain [   ]
   g) pursue [   ]

4. Find errors in the transcription of the consonant sounds in the following words. In each word there is one error, indicating an impossible pronunciation of that word for a native speaker of English of any variety. Make a correct transcription in the space provided after the word.

   a) mothball [maðbɔl] should be [maθbɔl]
   b) wives [wajvs] should be [   ]
   c) recommend [rɛcəmɛnd] should be [   ]
   d) treasure [trɛzər] should be [   ]
   e) shipping [ʃɪppɪŋ] should be [   ]
   f) conniving [kənnajvɪŋ] should be [   ]
   g) resounding [rəsawndɪŋ] should be [   ]

5. Find errors in the transcription of the vowel sounds in the following words. In each word there is one error, indicating an impossible pronunciation of

that word for a native speaker of English of any variety. Make a correct transcription in the space provided after the word.

a) minerals [minərəlz] should be [mɪnərəlz]
b) fishing [fiʃɪŋ] should be [   ]
c) regular [rɛgulər] should be [   ]
d) biennial [bajænɪəl] should be [   ]
e) couldn't [kudnt] should be [   ]
f) programming [programɪŋ] should be [   ]
g) football [futbɔl] should be [   ]

Reference

IPA Chart. (2015). Retrieved from http://www.internationalphoneticassociation.org/ content/ipa-chart, available under a Creative Commons Attribution-Sharealike 3.0 Unported License. Copyright © 2015 International Phonetic Association.

3 Phonology
The Patterning of Sounds

3.1 Introduction

Phonology is the study of how sounds pattern in a language. While phonetics is concerned with the physical production and perception of speech sounds, phonology describes the ways in which sounds function within a language to encode meaning. Phonological knowledge helps us to produce sounds that form meaningful utterances. For example, it helps us to choose the appropriate sound of the plural -*s* morpheme to turn singular nouns into plural nouns in English (e.g., [s] for *cups*, [z] for *spoons*, and [ɪz] for *dishes*), or the appropriate sound of the past tense -*ed* morpheme to form past tense verbs (e.g., [t] for *passed*, [d] for *reasoned*, and [ɪd] for *lasted*). For native speakers of English, knowing which sound to use in the formation of the plural noun or the past tense verb is largely subconscious (it is not so apparent for nonnative speakers of English, and this chapter will show how teachers can help students gain this knowledge). Phonology is about describing this subconscious knowledge that speakers have of their language.

In this chapter, we will learn that speakers and listeners of any language pay attention to contrastive sounds that signal a difference in meaning (i.e., phonemes) and ignore phonetically conditioned variation between non-contrastive sounds (i.e., allophones). We will see that what constitutes a phoneme is language-specific. For example, the difference between the vowels [i] and [ɪ] is crucial to English, as we can see from minimal pairs like *keen* [kin] and *kin* [kɪn]. But in Korean, this difference in pronunciation is not distinctive. A Korean speaker may pronounce the word for "long" as [kin] or [kɪn], and it will make no difference to the meaning.

When learning a second language, people naturally resort to their knowledge of their native language phonology. Thus, a Korean speaker may not always make a distinction between the vowels [i] and [ɪ] when pronouncing English words. This explains why many people speak a second language with an accent. We will review some strategies teachers can use to help students learn second language phonology and improve their pronunciation.

3.2 What Does It Mean When We Say We Know a Word?

Knowing a word means knowing both its sounds and its meaning. Most of the words in a language differ both in sounds and meaning. Consider the following words in English:

pat [pæt]	teal [til]	thigh [θaɪ]
bat [bæt]	deal [dil]	thy [ðaɪ]

Each word differs from the other words in both its sounds and meaning. Sometimes two words differ by just one sound. For example, the sounds of *pat* and *bat* are identical except for the initial consonant sounds. The *p* and *b* sounds can therefore distinguish or contrast words, and are called phonemes. **Phonemes** of a given language are heard by its native speakers as distinct sounds that result in a difference in meaning.

We see from the contrast between *teal* and *deal* and between *thigh* and *thy* that [t], [d], [θ], [ð] are also phonemes in English for the same reason—substituting a [d] for [t] or a [θ] for [ð] produces a different word. The difference between *pat* and *bat*, between *teal* and *deal*, and between *thigh* and *thy* are minimal (i.e., they are identical except for one sound that occurs in the same place in the word). For that reason, they are called **minimal pairs**. We can come up with more words that differ with *pat* and *bat* in the beginning consonant such as *mat, sat, fat*, and *vat*. These words form a **minimal set** with *pat* and *bat*. Likewise, we can form a minimal set by substituting the vowel sound in *pat*, as in *pet, pit, pot*, and *put*. We can form yet a different minimal set by substituting the final consonant in *pat*, as in *pad, pal, path*, and *pack*.

3.3 Phonemes and Allophones

In our discussion of voiceless stops in Chapter 2, we did not make a distinction between the *p* sound in the word *pit* from the *p* sound in the word *spit*. But try pronouncing these two words while holding a strip of paper in front of your lips and you will see (and hear) a clear difference between the two *p* sounds. When you say *pit*, a puff of air will push the paper. The paper will not move when you say *spit*. We call the *p* in *pit* **aspirated** and transcribe it using a small raised [ʰ] after the [p]. The *p* in *spit* is **unaspirated** and is transcribed with a regular [p]. Thus, *pit* is transcribed as [pʰɪt] and *spit* is transcribed as [spɪt].

After the release of the aspirated *p* in *pit* [pʰɪt], there is a brief delay before the start of voicing of the following vowel, [ɪ]. This lag in the onset of voicing is accompanied by release of air, giving rise to the puff of air (aspiration). In contrast, voicing of the vowel starts very soon after release of the unaspirated *p* in *spit* [spɪt]. There is a clear audible difference between the aspirated *p* and the unaspirated *p*. However, speakers of English typically perceive the [pʰ] in *pit* and the [p] in *spit* to be the same *p* sound. Why is this? This is because the difference between the two sounds is predictable and their occurrence can be determined by specific phonetic environments. Furthermore, changing one sound for the other will not change the meaning of the word.

To understand this point, let us examine some data. Table 3.1 lists examples of aspirated and unaspirated consonants in monosyllabic words (words made up of a single syllable). Notice that the sounds that have both aspirated and unaspirated varieties are all voiceless stops. The *t* in *tuck* and the *k* in *cone* are also aspirated voiceless stops, while the *t* in *stuck* and the *k* in *scone* are unaspirated voiceless stops.

Looking at Table 3.1, you will notice that all the aspirated stops occur at the beginning of the word while the unaspirated stops do not. But what happens when the word has more than one syllable? How do voiceless stops behave in words that have multiple syllables?

Let us consider some multisyllabic words in English such as *contain* [kən.tʰɛ́ɪn], *repeal* [rɪ.pʰíl], *articulate* [ar.tʰí.kjə.leɪt], *respect* [rɪ.spɛ́kt], *compass* [kʰám.pəs], and *marker* [már.kər] (note that the "." marks syllable boundaries while an acute accent [´] marks the primary stress in the word). When we examine these words, we notice that all the aspirated stops occur at the beginning of a syllable with a stressed vowel. The unaspirated stop, on the other hand, occurs in non-syllable-initial positions and in unstressed syllables. This observation leads us to the following phonological rule:

The phonemes /p/, /t/, and /k/ become [pʰ], [tʰ], and [kʰ] respectively when they occur at the beginning of a stressed (or, only) syllable. In non-syllable-initial positions or in non-stressed syllables, /p/, /t/, and /k/ are uttered as [p], [t], and [k] respectively.

Notice that where the aspirated *p* occurs, the unaspirated *p* does not, and where the unaspirated *p* occurs, the aspirated *p* does not. This mutual exclusivity makes it possible for us to determine when to use the aspirated *p* and when to use the unaspirated *p*. We call the aspirated *p* and the unaspirated *p*

Table 3.1 Monosyllabic English Words With Aspirated and Unaspirated Consonants

Aspirated	*Unaspirated*
paid [pʰeɪd]	spade [speɪd]
tuck [tʰʌk]	stuck [stʌk]
cone [kʰown]	scone [skown]

allophones of the /p/ phoneme. **Allophones** are predictable variants of one phoneme. In other words, the choice of which allophone to use is not random but can be predicted from examining the phonetic environment. Notice in the aforementioned rule that slashes / / are used to enclose phonemes and square brackets [ ] are used for allophones. The phoneme, /p/, is the representation of the sound in the mind of the English speaker while the allophones, [pʰ] and [p], are how that mental representation is produced in actual speech depending on the phonetic environment.

While native speakers of English know when to produce aspirated voiceless stops and when to produce unaspirated voiceless stops, they are not explicitly taught these rules. Rather, they acquire these rules subconsciously as children. But people who are learning English as a second language do not have this knowledge and need to learn the rule explicitly if they want to pronounce voiceless stops appropriately. This is where the ESL teacher would come in. By teaching the aspiration rule in English voiceless stops, teachers can help their students improve their pronunciation.

It is important to remember that phonological rules are language-specific. While the aspiration rule applies to English voiceless stops, the same rule does not apply to voiceless stops in other languages. In English, the aspirated *p* and the unaspirated *p* are allophones of the same phoneme, /p/. Therefore, if an ESL student were to pronounce *paid* as [pɛɪd] rather than [pʰɛɪd], it would sound a little "strange" but it would not result in a word with a different meaning. However, in languages such as Hindi or Korean, aspirated and unaspirated stops are separate phonemes (i.e., the use of one or the other results in difference in meaning). In these languages, making the distinction between aspirated and unaspirated stops is crucial because if you use the wrong sound, you may wind up saying something entirely different by mistake. Korean makes a three-way distinction in voiceless stops:

[t̬am] "sweat" (unaspirated, tense)
[tam] "fence" (slightly aspirated, lax)
[tʰam] "greed" (heavily aspirated)

This minimal triplet shows that [t̬], [t], and [tʰ] are separate phonemes in Korean that result in a difference in meaning depending on which one is used.

English speakers who are learning other languages should remember that while syllable-initial /p/, /t/, and /k/ are pronounced with strong aspiration in American English as [pʰ], [tʰ], and [kʰ], they are not produced with aspiration in many other languages. Those who wish to sound more "native-like" in languages like Spanish, for example, should pronounce the unaspirated versions of these consonants and use them only. Thus, Spanish words such as *casa* "house", *pero* "but", and *tostada* "toast" with voiceless stops in word-initial position should be pronounced as [kasa], [pɛro], [tostaða], and not as [kʰasa], [pʰɛro], and [tʰostʰada].

Voices From the Classroom 3.1 — Knowledge of Other Languages Comes in Handy When Teaching English Pronunciation

My knowledge of students' native languages helps me understand some of my students' pronunciation issues. In Arabic, [p] and [b] are allophones so Arabic speakers often say *labtob* for *laptop*. I tell my students both [p] and [b] are made the same way with the lips and mouth but that [b] vibrates in the throat. I have them put their fingers on the throat and feel the vibration as they practice saying the sounds [p] and [b] and then have them practice the sounds in words. I like to use mirrors and discuss mouth shapes when practicing pronunciation, especially for vowels. Lax vowels are rare in other languages so I have students watch as they make the [i] and [ɪ] with their mouth opening wider for [i]. Predicting what issues beginners will have helps me understand what they are trying to say. Likewise, warning students that certain sounds are hard for speakers of certain languages alerts them that they should try to focus on these sounds.

Hilary Reintges, Adult ESL Teacher

3.4 Natural Classes

In generating phonological rules, it is helpful to refer to the concept of natural classes. A **natural class** is a group of sounds in a language that share one or more articulatory or auditory property, to the exclusion of other sounds in that language. For example, consonants constitute a natural class to the exclusion of vowels. Similarly, voiced sounds form a natural class to the exclusion of voiceless sounds. The same principle applies to labial sounds vs. non-labial sounds, nasals vs. non-nasals, front vowels vs. non-front vowels, etc.

When trying to identify natural classes for consonants, look for what a group of consonants have in common in terms of voicing, place of articulation, and manner of articulation. When identifying natural classes for vowels, look for what the vowels have in common in terms of tongue height, front/back, tenseness, and lip rounding.

Natural classes are important because it is easier to learn a rule that applies to a whole class of sounds than to individual sounds. For example, in the previously discussed English aspiration rule, we saw that a natural class—namely, voiceless stops, /p/, /t/, and /k/—are affected by this phonological rule. Voiced stops and other classes of sounds are not affected by this rule. Natural classes help us to understand how sounds pattern in a language by allowing us to efficiently and economically describe how a whole group of sounds are affected by a variety of phonological processes.

Let us illustrate the significance of natural classes by way of two examples: Canadian Raising and Vowel Length in English.

3.4.1 Canadian Raising

Canadian Raising is a phonological rule in many dialects of North American English that changes the pronunciation of diphthongs, [aɪ] and [aʊ], to [ʌɪ] and [ʌʊ] respectively. It gets its name from a low vowel, [a], being raised to a mid vowel, [ʌ]. Speakers of these dialects would say *out and about* as [ʌʊt ən əbʌʊt] rather than [aʊt ən əbaʊt], and *bright light* as [brʌɪt lʌɪt] rather than [braɪt laɪt]. However, the pronunciation changes do not happen across the board to all words containing these diphthongs. Some words with these diphthongs retain the [aɪ] and [aʊ] pronunciation as in other dialects of English.

Our job as students of phonology is to determine when the change in the pronunciation occurs and when it does not. In other words, is the change in pronunciation governed by a phonological rule? If so, what is that rule? To answer this question, we need to examine words that are pronounced with [aɪ] and words that are pronounced with [ʌɪ] in these dialects of North American English.

Consider the following data. Notice that the left column has words that are pronounced with the diphthong [aɪ], and the right column, with the diphthong [ʌɪ].

[aɪ]	*[ʌɪ]*
rise [raɪz]	bite [bʌɪt]
time [taɪm]	bike [bʌɪk]
file [faɪl]	life [lʌɪf]
ninth [naɪnθ]	type [tʌɪp]

Based on these data, we can list the phonetic environments of the two diphthongs as follows. The "phonetic environment" typically means the sound that is immediately to the left and the sound that is immediately to the right of the sound in question. Notice that we use a dash (—) to stand for the sounds in question, [aɪ] and [ʌɪ]:

[aɪ]	*[ʌɪ]*
r—z	b—t
t—m	b—k
f—l	l—f
n—n	t—p

Look at the sounds that occur before [aɪ] in the left column and see if they form a natural class. In other words, look for what they have in common in terms of voicing, place of articulation, and manner of articulation. Then, look at the sounds to the right of [aɪ] and see what they have in common in terms of voicing, place of articulation, and manner of articulation. Now, look at the sounds to the left of [ʌɪ] and see if you can identify any natural classes. Finally, repeat the same process for the sounds to the right of [ʌɪ].

When we do this, we notice that the sounds that are immediately to the right of [aɪ] are all voiced consonants whereas the sounds that are immediately to the right of [ʌɪ] are all voiceless consonants. Voiced consonants and voiceless consonants are mutually exclusive categories (i.e., they form natural classes) and we can therefore say that the distribution of [aɪ] and [ʌɪ] is determined by the phonetic environment. In other words, we can predict when the diphthong /aɪ/ will be pronounced as [aɪ] and when it will be pronounced as [ʌɪ]. So, we can write a phonological rule that captures this fact as follows:

(1) [aɪ] occurs before a voiced consonant whereas [ʌɪ] occurs before a voiceless consonant.

We can also write the phonological rule in (1) in a different way, as (2):

(2) /aɪ/ becomes [ʌɪ] before a voiceless consonant.

Notice that (1) and (2) are the same rule written in different ways. While (1) shows that [aɪ] and [ʌɪ] are allophones of the same phoneme, (2) shows that /aɪ/ is the phonemic form of the diphthong, which is pronounced as [ʌɪ] before a voiceless consonant and [aɪ] before a voiced consonant.

Let us now consider words that contain [aʊ] and [ʌʊ] in dialects with Canadian Raising:

[aʊ]	*[ʌʊ]*
howl [haʊl]	about [əbʌʊt]
browse [braʊz]	house [hʌʊs]
cloud [klaʊd]	south [sʌʊθ]
pound [paʊnd]	clout [klʌʊt]

We can list the phonetic environments of these words as follows:

[aʊ]	*[ʌʊ]*
h—l	b—t
r—z	h—s
l—d	s—θ
p—n	l—t

Looking at the phonetic environments, we notice that the same rule applies to [aʊ] and [ʌʊ]—namely, that [aʊ] occurs before a voiced consonant whereas [ʌʊ] occurs before a voiceless consonant.

This analysis shows that the natural classes of voiced consonants vs. voiceless consonants elegantly describe the distribution of the two types of diphthongs in some dialects of North American English. The mutually exclusive nature of voiced consonants vs. voiceless consonants helps us predict when we will get the raised diphthongs, [ʌɪ] and [ʌʊ], and when we will not.

3.4.2 Vowel Length in English

Now, let us consider another example of allophonic variation—that of vowel length. The colon [:] placed after [ɪ] in the words in the right column means that the vowel is long.

[ɪ]	*[ɪː]*
hiss [hɪs]	his [hɪːz]
rich [rɪtʃ]	ridge [rɪːdʒ]
trick [trɪk]	trig [trɪːg]
hit [hɪt]	hid [hɪːd]
slip [slɪp]	slim [slɪːm]

We can list the phonetic environments of the two sounds in question as follows:

[ɪ]	*[ɪː]*
h—s	h—z
r—tʃ	r—dʒ
r—k	r—g
h—t	h—d
l—p	l—m

When we consider the phonetic environments of [ɪ] and [ɪː], we notice that the sounds that are immediately to the right of [ɪ] are all voiceless consonants whereas the sounds immediately to the right of [ɪː] are all voiced consonants. Therefore, we can say that the distribution of [ɪ] and [ɪː] is phonologically conditioned. In other words, we can predict when the phoneme /ɪ/, will be pronounced as [ɪ] and when it will be pronounced as [ɪː]. So, we can write a phonological rule that captures this fact as follows:

(3) [ɪ] occurs before a voiceless consonant while [ɪː] occurs before a voiced consonant.

We can also write the phonological rule in (3) in a different way, as (4):

(4) /ɪ/ becomes [ɪ:] before a voiced consonant.

Notice that (4) shows that /ɪ/ is the phonemic form of the vowel, which is uttered as [ɪ:] before a voiced consonant and [ɪ] before a voiceless consonant. Therefore, [ɪ] and [ɪ:] are allophones of the phoneme /ɪ/. As explained earlier, the phoneme /ɪ/ is the representation of the sound in the mind of the English speaker while the allophones [ɪ] and [ɪ:] are how that mental representation is produced in actual speech depending on the phonetic environment.

Vowel length is allophonic in most dialects of English. That is, a monosyllabic word that ends in a voiceless consonant will be shorter than the same word that ends in a voiced consonant. You can see this in a minimal pair such as *pat* and *pad*. Try saying these two words and you will notice that the vowel [æ] in [pæd] is slightly longer than the vowel [æ] in [pæt]. The same rule applies to *neat* and *need*, to *but* and *bud*, and even to diphthongs like *write* and *ride*, and *mouth* (noun) and *mouth* (verb). Words that end in a voiced consonant have vowels that are slightly longer than those that end in a voiceless consonant.

The vowel lengthening rule applies to the speech of all speakers of English regardless of style or rate of speaking. While the length differences are ever so small and not very easy to notice, they are nonetheless an important part of a native accent. Not applying the rule of vowel lengthening would make someone sound like a nonnative speaker of English. Also, keep in mind that vowel length here is used differently than the notion of long vowels and short vowels in phonics (see Chapter 2); vowel length here is literally the time each vowel lasts, while phonics uses long and short vowels to refer to two different vowels in English, like the long i (as in *bite*) and the short i (as in *bit*).

More importantly, not getting the right vowel length can interfere with communication. For example, the final stops, [t] and [d], in *pat* and *pad* are often unreleased. That is, the final stop has no audible release. Unreleased stops are marked by a raised [˺] after the stop, as in [pæt˺] and [pæ:d˺]. We see instances of unreleased stops in the first consonant of clusters in words such as *doctor* [dɑk˺tər] and *kept* [kɛp˺t].

When the final stop in words like *pat* and *pad* is unreleased, the length of the preceding vowel plays a crucial role in communicating to the listener which word was meant by the speaker. The slightly longer vowel in [pæ:d˺] will signal to the listener that the word *pad* was meant by the speaker and not the word *pat* [pæt˺]. Without an audible release in the final stop, the only clue that the listener has is the length of the preceding vowel.

Not getting the right vowel length is a common pronunciation problem for many ESL students. Few students know that there is a difference between the vowels in *pat* and *pad*. Here again, the ESL teacher can help students produce the right vowel length by explicitly teaching the vowel lengthening rule in English. Teachers can do exercises involving minimal pairs (e.g., cap/cab, heat/heed, muck/mug, ate/aid, bright/bride). By exaggerating vowel length differences in minimal pairs such as these, teachers can sensitize students to accurately perceive and produce words in English.

3.5 Phonological Processes

Phonological rules may be obligatory or optional. **Obligatory rules** apply in the speech of all speakers of a language or dialect having the rule, regardless of style or rate of speaking. Canadian Raising and Vowel Length in English, which we discussed previously, are obligatory rules that apply in the speech of all speakers of those dialects. On the other hand, the unreleased final stop is an optional rule that sometimes applies in casual speech. **Optional rules** may or may not apply in any given utterance and are responsible for variation in speech.

Another optional rule in English is **deletion** in unstressed syllables. Deletion rules eliminate a sound, frequently in unstressed syllables and in casual speech. Deletion is common in fast speech because it saves time and effort for the speaker. So, the sentence *I want him to see this* may be said either as [aɪ wənt hɪm tə si ðɪs] in careful speech, or as [aɪ wən ɪm tə si ðɪs] in more casual speech. The voiceless stop, /t/, after a nasal at the end of the word *want* is often deleted, especially when the final stop is unreleased. Sounds like /h/ that are not very noticeable are often deleted because speakers can save time and effort by eliminating them without sacrificing meaning.

In addition, an unstressed vowel [ə], is often deleted when the next syllable is stressed in fast speech, as shown in Table 3.2.

As deleting sounds can make speech production easier in these examples, **insertion** of sounds can accomplish the same goal in others. Insertion is especially helpful when producing two neighboring sounds that have very different phonetic features. For example, the words *warmth, tenth*, and *length* are typically pronounced [wɔrmθ], [tɛnθ], and [lɛŋθ]. In casual speech, however, speakers may insert a [p] between the [m] and the [θ] and pronounce the word [wɔrmpθ]. Similarly, a [t] may be inserted between [n] and [θ] to produce [tɛntθ], and a [k] may be inserted between [ŋ] and [θ] to produce [lɛŋkθ].

There is an articulatory explanation to this process. The insertion of a voiceless stop consonant makes it easier for the articulators to transition from a voiced nasal to a voiceless fricative in these words. Table 3.3 describes [m] and [θ] in terms of voicing, place, and manner of articulation. Notice that these

Table 3.2 Deletion of Vowel [ə] in Unstressed Syllables

	Slow speech	Fast speech
corruption	[kʰərˈʌpʃən]	[kɹˈʌpʃən]
ferocious	[fərˈóʊʃəs]	[fɹˈóʊʃəs]
ballistic	[bəlístɪk]	[blístɪk]

Note: The [ˌ] placed below [r] in [kɹˈʌpʃən] and [fɹóʊʃəs] denotes devoicing.

two sounds have no common feature—they are very different sounds. Articulatorily speaking, it is not very easy to go from [m] to [θ] in quick succession.

Now look at Table 3.4, which lists the features for [m], [p], and [θ]. Notice that as the articulators go from [m] to [p] to [θ], there is overlapping place and voicing that the inserted sound, [p], has in common with the preceding and the following sound. In other words, the transition is more gradual than if the articulators were to go directly from [m] to [θ].

Aside from those explained so far, there are a few phonological processes that are very common in the world's languages.

One of the most common phonological processes found in many of the world's languages is assimilation. Quite simply, **assimilation** causes a sound to become more like a neighboring sound in terms of one or more of its phonetic characteristics. Assimilation occurs mainly for ease of articulation; that is, assimilation makes it easier to move the articulators to produce different sounds consecutively in fluent speech.

In Table 3.2, we saw that [r], a typically voiced sound, became voiceless after voiceless consonants, [k] and [f], in fast speech. This process is called **devoicing**. Liquids and glides after voiceless consonants in English words such as *play* [pl̥eɪ], *prod* [pr̥ad], and *cure* [kj̥ur] are often devoiced. Devoicing is a kind of assimilation because the lack of voicing in the [p] and [k] sounds spreads to [l], [r], and [j], making these normally voiced sounds voiceless. Speaking in terms of articulatory phonetics, devoicing happens because the vocal folds do not start vibrating immediately after the release of the voiceless consonant closure.

Table 3.3 [m] and [θ] Described in Terms of Voicing, Place, and Manner

	Voicing	Place	Manner
[m]	Voiced	Bilabial	Nasal
[θ]	Voiceless	Interdental	Fricative

Table 3.4 [m], [p], and [θ] Described in Terms of Voicing, Place, and Manner

	Voicing	Place	Manner
[m]	Voiced	**Bilabial**	Nasal
[p]	**Voiceless**	**Bilabial**	Stop
[θ]	**Voiceless**	Interdental	Fricative

Voices From the Classroom 3.2—Teaching the Different Pronunciations of the -*ed* Ending

When teaching past tense, I use phonology to teach the different pro-nunciations of the -*ed* ending. For this lesson, I explain the difference between voiced and voiceless sounds, asking students to touch their throats as we go through different sounds together so they can feel their vocal cords vibrating or not. Then, in groups, they receive a stack of cards, each with three words with -*ed* on them (for example, one card might have *asked, filled,* and *wanted*). Together, students decide on the pronunciation for each word, label the words with /t/, /d/, or /ɪd/, and practice saying them. It's very rewarding, as a teacher, to walk around and see students touching their vocal cords, trying out the different pro-nunciations—and getting them right based on their new understanding of voiced and voiceless sounds.

Erica Ashton, ESL Teacher

Other than **voicing assimilation**, assimilation for place and manner of articulation is also widespread in the world's languages. An example of **place assimilation** is the pronunciation of the prefix *un-* in English. Words like *unbeatable, unjust,* and *uncut* are often pronounced [əmbiɾəbl̩], [ənd͡ʒʌst], and [əŋkʌt]. The nasal /n/ is often pronounced as a bilabial nasal, [m], before a bilabial sound, as in [əmbiɾəbl̩], and as a velar nasal, [ŋ], before a velar sound, as in [əŋkʌt]. The nasal stays as an alveolar nasal, [n], before a post-alveolar affricate, [d͡ʒ], in [ənd͡ʒʌst]. Thus, when an alveolar nasal immediately pre-cedes a bilabial consonant, assimilation causes it to become a bilabial nasal. When it immediately precedes a velar consonant, the same process causes the alveolar nasal to become a velar nasal. In other words, the nasal is assimilated to the place of articulation of the following consonant.

An example of **manner assimilation** can be seen in nasalization of vowels before a nasal consonant, as shown in Table 3.5. Nasalization of a vowel before a nasal consonant is caused by speakers anticipating the lowering of the velum in preparation for a nasal sound. The result is that the preceding sound takes on the nasality of the following nasal consonant. Nasalized vowels occur only before nasal consonants in English syllables and are therefore predictable vari-ants (allophones) of vowel phonemes.

However, as shown by minimal pairs in Table 3.6, nasal and oral vowels contrast in French, that is, they are separate phonemes in that language. The distribution of oral vs. nasal vowels is not determined by the phonetic envi-ronment since the oral vowels and their nasal counterparts occur in the same environment.

Table 3.5 Vowel Nasalization in English

Oral vowels	Nasalized vowels
lead [lid]	lean [lĩn]
sack [sæk]	sang [sæ̃ŋ]
face [feɪs]	fame [fẽɪm]

Table 3.6 How Oral and Nasal Vowels Contrast in French

Oral vowels	Nasal vowels
gras [grɑ] "fatty"	grand [grɑ̃] "tall"
beau [bo] "beautiful"	bon [bõ] "good"
paix [pɛ] "peace"	pain [pɛ̃] "bread"

The opposite of assimilation is **dissimilation**, in which a sound becomes less like a neighboring sound in terms of one of more of its phonetic characteristics. Compared to assimilation, dissimilation is a much rarer phonological process. However, when it does occur, it frequently serves the purpose of achieving clearer communication by breaking up sounds that are too similar. For example, in English, the word *fifths* [fɪfθs] ends in a consonant cluster made up of three consecutive fricatives. Some speakers pronounce this word as [fɪfts], breaking up the sequence of three fricatives with a stop.

Strengthening is a phonological process that makes sounds stronger. Aspiration of voiceless stops in English, discussed earlier in this chapter, is an example of strengthening. Aspirated stops are stronger sounds than unaspirated stops because the lag in the onset of voicing in aspirated stops is accompanied by a puff of air, which gives the sound a stronger quality.

The opposite of strengthening is **weakening**, a process by which sounds become weaker. **Flapping** is an example of weakening. Like a stop, a flap involves completely obstructing the oral cavity. But the duration of obstruction is much shorter than that of a stop. American English has an alveolar flap, [ɾ], which involves the tip of the tongue quickly striking the roof of the mouth and returning to its rest position. The flap occurs as the middle sound in the words, *butter* [bʌɾər], *writer* [raɪɾər], *ladder* [læɾər], and *tidal* [taɪɾəl]. Notice that in these words, a *t* or a *d* sound becomes [ɾ] when it occurs between two vowels—specifically, after a stressed vowel and before an unstressed vowel. The flap is a weaker sound than [t] or [d] because it is shorter in duration and obstructs less air. Notice that when [t] changes to [ɾ] in these words, it involves voicing assimilation: [t], a voiceless sound, takes on the voicing of its surrounding vowels by becoming [ɾ], a voiced sound.

Finally, **metathesis** is a phonological process that reorders sounds. In many cases, sounds metathesize to make words easier to pronounce or easier to understand. In some dialects of English, for example, the word *ask* is pronounced as *aks*. Some English-speaking adults pronounce *prescription, introduce,* and *cavalry* as *perscription, interduce,* and *calvary*. In each of these instances, metathesis facilitates the pronunciation of consonant cluster sequences.

3.6 Syllables

So far, we have discussed phonemes and allophones, and have seen that allophonic variation is often conditioned by neighboring sounds. We turn now to a different unit of phonological representation, namely, the syllable. Just as phonemes and allophones are part of speakers' knowledge, syllables are also part of speakers' knowledge about how sounds pattern in their language.

In any given language, a word is composed of one or more syllables, and a **syllable** is in turn composed of one or more phonemes. Every syllable has a **nucleus**, or a vowel. The nucleus may be preceded by one or more consonants called the **onset** and followed by one or more consonants called the **coda**. The nucleus and coda together are called the **rhyme**.

Figures 3.1 through 3.3 show the structures of monosyllabic English words, *ah, ark,* and *shark*. Notice that a syllable can be made up of just a vowel nucleus (as in *ah*), or nucleus and coda (as in *ark*), or onset, nucleus, and coda (as in *shark*).

Whenever native speakers of a language count syllables in a word, they demonstrate their knowledge of the syllable as a phonological unit. For example, English speakers intuitively know that the word *composition* [kam.pə.zı.ʃən] has four syllables because it has four vowels that serve as syllable nuclei ("." marks syllable divisions). Children learn from an early age that the nucleus

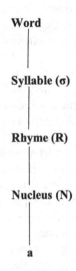

Figure 3.1 English Syllable Structure for *"Ah"*

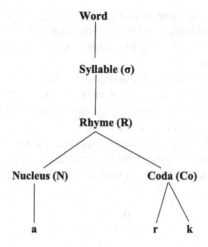

Figure 3.2 English Syllable Structure for *"Ark"*

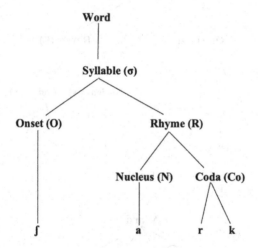

Figure 3.3 English Syllable Structure for *"Shark"*

and the coda of the final syllable in rhyming words are identical, as shown in the following nursery rhyme:

Humpty Dumpty sat on a w<u>all</u> /ɔl/
Humpty Dumpty had a great f<u>all</u> /ɔl/
All the king's horses and all the king's m<u>en</u> /ɛn/
Couldn't put Humpty together ag<u>ain</u> /ɛn/

Just as what constitutes a phoneme is language-specific, what constitutes a syllable is also language-specific. Each language has its own definition of what may be considered a syllable in that language. Figure 3.4 shows the syllable structure of a monosyllabic word in English, *sprint*. The vowel, /ɪ/, constitutes the nucleus, while the remaining five sounds /s/, /p/, /r/, /n/, and /t/ are part of either the onset or the coda.

While *sprint* is a monosyllabic word in English, when the Japanese borrow the word, *sprint*, it is pronounced as *su.pu.rin.to* with four syllables (see Figure 3.5). This is because Japanese syllable structure does not allow consonant clusters in the onset or in the coda, as does English. Therefore, when borrowing words from other languages, Japanese speakers break up consonant clusters into separate consonants by inserting a vowel after each consonant. Notice that the only coda that is allowed in Japanese is /n/.

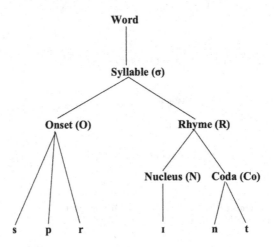

Figure 3.4 English Syllable Structure for *"Sprint"*

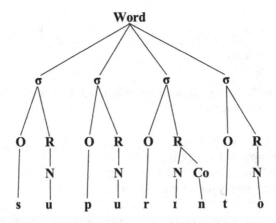

Figure 3.5 Japanese Syllable Structure for *"Sprint"*

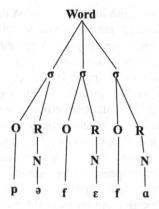

Figure 3.6 English Syllable Structure for "*Pfeffer*" [pəfɛfɑ]

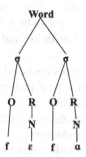

Figure 3.7 English Syllable Structures for "*Pfeffer*" [fɛfɑ]

Just as a Japanese-speaking learner of English would have difficulty pronouncing *sprint* as one syllable, an English speaker who is learning German would have difficulty pronouncing a word like *pfeffer* /pfɛfɑ/ "pepper" since the /pf/ sequence is not a permissible onset for a syllable in English. Thus, many English speakers would pronounce this German word as either [pəfɛfɑ] by inserting an extra vowel, or as [fɛfɑ] by deleting the initial consonant (see Figures 3.6 and 3.7).

3.7 How to Help Students Improve Their Pronunciation in a Second Language

When trying to help students improve their pronunciation in a second language, it is important to remember that second language pronunciation problems are often rooted in differences between what constitutes a phoneme or a syllable in the student's native language versus the target language. Consequently, it is helpful for teachers to become familiar with the phonology of the student's native language.

The Internet provides a wealth of information on the sound inventories of the world's languages. Teachers can do a quick search using key words such as *Spanish phonemic inventory, Arabic phonology*, or *Finnish vowels* and find articles written on these topics. Wikipedia provides an easy reference on the consonant and vowel inventories of many languages.

Let's see how a study of the phonemic inventory of students' native language can help teachers address students' pronunciation difficulties. A quick look at the Castilian Spanish consonant phoneme inventory (see Table 3.7) reveals that this language does not have /v/. Although the letter *v* is used in Spanish writing, the *v* sound does not exist in most dialects of Spanish. Therefore, you might hear Spanish speakers substitute the *v* sound with a *b* sound in English and say *bat* for *vat*, and *Boyd* for *void*. They may also substitute /v/ with /β/, a voiced labial fricative and say [seβən] for *seven*. [β] is an allophone of the phoneme /b/ that occurs between vowels.

Another observation from the Spanish consonant inventory is that it does not have a voiceless palatal fricative, /ʃ/, which suggests that Spanish speakers may have difficulty pronouncing words with /ʃ/ in English. In fact, many Spanish speakers will substitute /ʃ/ with /tʃ/, and pronounce *shock* as *chock* and *wish* as *witch*.

What can teachers do to help Spanish-speaking students accurately produce sounds like /v/ and /ʃ/ that do not exist in their native language? First, teachers can explain how the *v* sound is produced by showing how the upper teeth touch the lower lip and how the air passes through the narrow opening to produce the turbulent noise heard in the production of /v/. Another way to approach this is to draw students' attention to the fact that pronouncing /v/ involves simply adding voicing to /f/, which they already know how to produce. Teachers might have students place the tip of their fingers on their throat while saying /f/ and /v/ alternately. They can explain that both these sounds are produced in the same way in the mouth and that the only difference between /f/ and /v/ is the absence or presence of voicing.

As for /ʃ/, even though it is not a phoneme in many dialects of Spanish, Spanish speakers can nonetheless produce this sound. Teachers can have students practice saying "shhh" as if telling someone to be quiet. Then, students

Table 3.7 Castilian Spanish Consonant Phoneme Inventory

	Labial	*Dental*	*Alveolar*	*Palatal*	*Velar*
Stop	p b	t d		tʃ	k g
Fricative	f		s	j	x
Nasal	m		n	ɲ	
Lateral			l		
Flap			ɾ		
Trill			r		

Source: Adapted from: Martínez-Celdrán et al., 2003

can add different vowel nuclei and coda to form words like *shhhock, shh-hip, shhhine,* or add different onsets and vowels to form words like *wishhh, mashhh, lushhh.*

When addressing pronunciation problems, teachers will want to exaggerate the differences in articulation between the sounds they are trying to contrast, using slower tempo and repetition to help students hear and feel the differences. As discussed in Chapter 2, teachers may also use a variety of teaching tools such as lollipops and mirrors to help students see the position and shape of the articulators (lips, teeth, tongue).

English has a particularly large inventory of vowel phonemes compared with most other languages in the world. This causes problems for students whose native languages have far fewer vowels. For example, the tense/lax distinction found in English vowels does not exist in many other languages. Thus, many ESL students will pronounce *deep* and *dip* in the same way and *coat* and *caught* in the same way. One strategy that works well involves doing exercises with minimal pairs such as the following:

/i/	/ɪ/
seat	sit
heed	hid
green	grin
steal	still

After practicing with minimal pairs in isolation, teachers can have students create sentences using the words in minimal pairs (e.g., "When invited to a party, don't <u>sit</u> in the most important <u>seat</u>" or "The big <u>green</u> monster had a wide <u>grin</u> on his face") and have students practice reading them accurately with a partner.

Further Reading

Avery, P., & Ehrlich, S. (1992). *Teaching American English pronunciation.* Oxford: Oxford University Press.

Graham, C. (2001). *Jazz Chants old and new: Student book* (2nd ed.). Oxford: Oxford University Press.

Exercises

1. Transcribe the following words phonetically. Then circle all words that form a minimal pair with *sap* /sæp/.

lap	cop	tab	tap	hope	tan	tip	top	cone
tar	zap	sip	team	map	tow	rap	nine	tad

2. Flapping: When do /d/ and /t/ become [ɾ] in American English? Examine the following data and determine the phonological rule. Note that in the following transcriptions, an acute accent ['] marks the primary stress in the word.

/t/ or /d/	/ɾ/
sandy [sǽndi]	pity [píɾi]
attention [ətɛ́nʃən]	magnetic [mægnɛ́ɾɪk]
tainted [téɪntɪd]	beauty [bjúɾi]
atone [ətóʊn]	ladle [léɪɾl̩]
compete [kəmpít]	daughter [dɔ́ɾər]
disdain [dɪsdéɪn]	udder [ʌ́ɾər]

3. Consider the distribution of [s] and [ʃ] in Korean in the following words. [ɯ] is a high back unrounded vowel.

saram "person"	ʃidʒaŋ "market"
suhak "mathematics"	ʃihʌm "test"
sʌnsɛŋ "teacher"	ʃinpal "shoe"
sɯmul "twenty"	ʃilsɯp "training"
kasu "singer"	kaʃi "thorn"

Based on these data, are [s] and [ʃ] allophones of the same phoneme or allophones of different phonemes? If they are allophones of the same phoneme, state their distribution.

4. Consider the distribution of [r] and [l] in Korean in the following words and determine whether these two sounds are allophones of one phoneme or of different phonemes.

baram "wind"	paltʰop "toenail"
kirin "giraffe"	sʌnpul "advance payment"
noritʌ "playground"	kalmang "craving"
suri "repair"	pʰilsu "necessary"
harapʌdʒi "grandfather"	halmʌni "grandmother"

If [r] and [l] are allophones of the same phoneme, which is the more basic form? How do you know?

5. Consider the distribution of [t], [ts], and [tʃ] in the following Japanese words and determine whether these three sounds are allophones of one phoneme or of different phonemes. Note that [ts] is an alveolar affricate and should be taken as a single symbol. Similarly, [tʃ] is an alveopalatal

affricate and should be taken as a single symbol. If the three sounds in question are allophones of the same phoneme, state the phonological rule.

tabemono "food"	tsukue "desk"
tʃigau "wrong"	todana "cupboard
tomodatʃi "friend"	tenki "weather"
totemo "very"	tsukuru "to make"
tʃikatetsu "subway"	tʃitʃi "father"
tokubetsu "special"	tsumori "plan"

6. Consider the distribution of [b], [d], [g], and [β], [ð], [ɣ] in the following Spanish data. [β] is a voiced bilabial fricative, [ð] is a voiced dental fricative, and [ɣ] is a voiced velar fricative. [b] and [β] are allophones of the same phoneme, as are [d] and [ð], as well as [g] and [ɣ]. State a rule that describes the conditioning environments for each pair.

[laðrar]	"to bark"	[kaða]	"each"	[doβle]	"double"
[boka]	"mouth"	[beβo]	"I drink"	[nombre]	"name"
[toðo]	"all"	[teŋgo]	"I have"	[tjenda]	"shop"
[graβaðor]	"recording"	[amiɣo]	"friend"	[siɣlo]	"century"

7. Consider the distribution of palatal affricates, [tʃ], [tʃʰ], [dʒ], and [dʒʰ], in the following data from Gujarati, a language spoken in the Indian state of Gujarat. [tʃʰ] is a voiceless aspirated palatal affricate and [dʒʰ] is a voiced aspirated palatal affricate. Determine if the four are allophones of the same phoneme or of separate phonemes. If they are allophones of the same phoneme, state a rule that describes the distribution. If they are allophones of separate phonemes, give a minimal set.

[tʃəl]	"walk"	[tʃidʒʰ]	"thing"	[dʒiɳɖgi]	"life"
[səmədʒ]	"understand"	[dʒəl]	"water"	[dʒʰəndə]	"flag"
[bidʒu]	"second"	[fĩtʃko]	"swing"	[dʒʰəl]	"glimmer"
[ekədʒ]	"one"	[tʃʰəl]	"deceit"	[tʃʰətri]	"umbrella"

Reference

Martínez-Celdrán, E., Fernández-Planas, A. M., & Carrera-Sabaté, J. (2003). Castilian Spanish. *Journal of the International Phonetic Association*, 33(2), 255–259.

4 Morphology
The Analysis of Words

4.1 Introduction

So far in this book, we have seen how individual sounds are produced (Chapter 2), and how sounds pattern within a language to form meaningful utterances (Chapter 3). In this chapter, we proceed to examining a slightly larger linguistic unit—words. Words are a crucial part of our mental grammars. Without knowledge of words, we would not be able to get our meanings across to other people. Unlike phonemes and syllables, which operate only at the level of sounds, words carry meaning in addition to sounds. Words are also permanently stored in a speaker's mental dictionary called **lexicon**. This permanence distinguishes words from phrases and sentences, which are pieced together with words as needed and then discarded when the need for them disappears (we will discuss sentence structure in Chapter 5). Quite simply, words are the building blocks of communication.

What is a word? What does it mean when we say we know a word? Knowing a word means knowing both its sounds and its meaning. Every speaker of English knows that *measure* is an English word, as are *measurement, measuring, measurable*, and *immeasurable*. However, even though *street* is an English word, English speakers know that they cannot say any of the following: *streetment, streeting, streetable, instreetable*. How do English speakers know that adding *-able* to *measure* results in another word, but adding *-able* to *street* does not? Morphology tries to capture this knowledge, which is largely subconscious.

Morphology is the study of the internal structure of words—how words are formed and what their relationships to other words are in the same language. It describes which meaningful pieces of language can be combined to form words and what the effects of such combinations are on the meaning or the grammatical function of the resulting word. For example, adding *-able* to *measure* modifies the grammatical function of *measure*, a verb, to an adjective, and it does so in the same way when attached to *do (doable)*, or *manage (manageable)*. Similarly, adding *re-* to *type* changes the meaning of *type* to indicate repetition, and it does so in the same way when added to *generate (regenerate)*, or *furbish (refurbish)*.

The average six-year-old child knows about 13,000 words. If the child produced her first word at the age of two, that would mean that she has learned

3,250 words a year, an average of nine words a day. It is also estimated that the average high school graduate knows about 60,000 words. That would mean that between the ages of six and eighteen, the student has learned 47,000 words, or about 3,900 words a year, an average of about ten words a day. This stock of words constitutes the mental dictionary that the student has internalized as part of acquiring her language. The student knows that she can create and understand countless other words by applying general rules to the entries in her mental lexicon.

In this chapter, we will analyze word structure by identifying each of the components and classifying them in terms of their contribution to the meaning and function of the larger word. We will see how words are formed in different languages, and how they are marked differently to show grammatical concepts such as number, tense, person, gender, and case. This chapter will show how knowledge of the principles of word formation can facilitate students' learning of new vocabulary and what teachers can do to help students acquire this knowledge.

4.2 Morphemes

The most important part of the word is the **morpheme**, the smallest linguistic unit with a meaning or a grammatical function. Morphemes are important because all languages use them as building blocks to construct words. The word *teacher*, for example, consists of two morphemes: *teach* (with the meaning of "give instruction in") and *-er* (which indicates that the whole word functions as a noun with the meaning "one who teaches"). Similarly, the word *schools* is composed of the morphemes *school* (with the meaning of "an institution where instruction is given") and *-s* (with the meaning "more than one").

Some words are made up of a single morpheme. Such words are said to be **simple words**. For example, the word *happy* cannot be divided into smaller parts that carry information about its meaning or function. Thus, the word *happy* consists of a single morpheme. In contrast, the word *impersonal* is made up of three morphemes, *im-person-al*. Words that contain two or more morphemes like *impersonal* are said to be **complex words**. It is important to not confuse morphemes with syllables. The word *happy* [hæ.pi] is one morpheme but has two syllables. The word *impersonal* [ɪm.pʌr.sə.nəl] is composed of three morphemes but has four syllables (note that the "." in the phonetic transcriptions marks syllable boundaries). Remember that a morpheme is the smallest linguistic unit with a meaning or a grammatical function.

Complex words typically consist of a root morpheme and one or more affixes. The **root** is the primary lexical unit of a word that carries the most significant aspects of semantic content and cannot be reduced into smaller parts. Roots typically belong to a lexical category such as noun (*man, nation, color, tree*), verb (*teach, form, make, think*), adjective (*honest, small, kind, quick*), or preposition (*about, in, to, from*).

Unlike roots, however, **affixes** do not belong to a lexical category. An affix that is attached to the front of the root is called a **prefix** (*dis-* in *dishonest*, *un-* in *uncertain*), whereas an affix that is attached to the end of the root is called a **suffix** (*-ful* in *beautiful*, *-ly* in *quickly*). Some words have multiple affixes attached to them. For example, the word *internationalizing* has a prefix (*inter-*) and three suffixes (*-al*, *-ize*, and *-ing*) attached to the root (*nation*).

Although many languages use prefixes and suffixes, a fewer number of languages also have **infixes**, affixes that are inserted into existing morphemes. For example, in Indonesian, the infix *-em-* is inserted after the first consonant in the root to create new words. Thus, *cemerlang* ("brilliant") is derived from *cerlang* ("luminous"), and *gemetar* ("to tremble") is derived from *getar* ("to vibrate").

Some languages also have **circumfixes**, morphemes that are attached to the front and the end of the root to form new words. In Malay, the circumfix *ke—an* is attached to adjectives to form nouns meaning "the state of (the adjective)". Thus, *kebaratan* ("the state of being west"), *ketimuran* ("the state of being east"), and *kebesaran* ("the state of being big") are derived from *barat* ("west"), *timur* ("east"), and *besar* ("big"). Circumfixes are different from prefixes and suffixes because both the front and end components need to be attached to the root for it to work.

4.3 Classifying Morphemes

There are mainly two kinds of morphemes. A morpheme that can stand alone as a word is called a **free morpheme**, whereas a morpheme that can only occur in words attached to other morphemes is called a **bound morpheme**. Most roots in English are free morphemes, although a limited number of roots (*ept* in *inept*, *mit* in *remit*) are bound morphemes and must combine with another morpheme to be an acceptable word.

Free morphemes can be further divided into content morphemes and function morphemes. This is shown in the left column in Table 4.1. **Content morphemes** carry meaning as opposed to merely perform a grammatical function, and constitute the major part of the vocabulary (e.g., nouns, verbs, adjectives, and adverbs). Content morphemes constitute what's called an **open class**, a lexical category into which new words are often introduced.

For instance, a lot of **loan words** (words that have been borrowed from other languages) tend to be nouns and belong to the category of open class. In English, loan words include terms that refer to foods (*smorgasbord, wok, satay*), popular culture (*paparazzi, karaoke, bikini*), and politics (*apartheid, realpolitik, pogrom*). As people from different cultures come into contact with one another, more and more words get added to the lexicon through borrowing. In addition, newly coined computer-related terms (*download, hyperlink, RAM, realtime*) also belong to the category of open class, as do existing words that have taken on additional meanings in online contexts (*friend, unfriend, ping*).

Function morphemes, on the other hand, provide information about the grammatical relationships between words in a sentence (e.g., articles, conjunctions, prepositions, and pronouns). Function morphemes constitute a **closed class**, a lexical category in which members are fairly rigidly established and additions are made very rarely.

The right column in Table 4.1 shows that bound morphemes can also be further divided into derivational morphemes and inflectional morphemes. **Derivational morphemes**, when combined with a root, change either the meaning or the part of speech of the word. Derivational morphemes in English are content morphemes and include both prefixes and suffixes. Table 4.2 provides some additional examples of derivational morphemes in English. Derivational morphemes have the following properties:

a) Change the part of speech and/or the meaning of a word (e.g., *-ment* in *statement, re-* in *rewrite*).

b) Are not required by syntax (e.g., The use of *un-* in *unhappy* changes the meaning of the sentence *He is unhappy* but is not required to make the sentence grammatical).

c) Are selective about what they can combine with (e.g., we can add *-hood* to *brother* to get *brotherhood*, but we cannot add *-hood* to *friend* to get **friendhood*). Note that the linguistic notation, "*", in front of *friendhood* indicates that this particular form is not acceptable.

d) Are typically attached before inflectional suffixes (e.g., *-ment* in *statement-s* must be added before *-s*).

Table 4.1 The Relationship Between Free and Bound Morphemes and Content and Function Morphemes in English

	Free Morphemes	*Bound Morphemes*
Content Morphemes	**_Open Class_** Nouns (*cat, tree, street, envy*) Verbs (*go, run, play, state*) Adjectives (*big, small, happy*) Adverbs (*fast, often, very*)	**_Bound Roots_** (*ept* in *inept, mit* in *remit,* *huckle* in *huckleberry*) **_Derivational Affixes_** Prefixes: (*re-, un-, dis-, inter-* as in: *rewrite, undo, dishonest,* *intercede*) Suffixes: (*-al, -ize, -ness, -ship* as in: *national, humanize,* *happiness, friendship*)
Function Morphemes	**_Closed Class_** Articles (*the, a, an*) Conjunctions (*and, or, but, so*) Prepositions (*in, on, above, beside*) Pronouns (*I, me, you, he, she, their*)	**_Inflectional Affixes_** All Suffixes: (*-s, -ed, -ing,* *-er, -est* as in: *books, played, singing,* *happier, happiest*)

Table 4.2 Some Derivational Affixes in English

Affix	Meaning	Examples
Prefixes:		
a-, an-	without	amoral, anaerobic, acellular
anti-	opposite of	anticlimax, antiseptic, antihero, antidepressant
circum-	around	circumference, circumnavigate, circumvent
dis-	not	disagree, disappear, discontinue, disobey
il-, im-, in-, ir-	not, without	illegal, impossible, inconsiderate, irresponsible
inter-	between, among	international, interstellar, intercede, intersect, intervene
post-	after, behind	postmortem, postscript, postoperative
un-	not, opposite of	unfinished, unfriendly, unskilled, unfair
Suffixes:		
-able, -ible	capable of being	abominable, credible, presentable, understandable
-al	pertaining to	emotional, grammatical, regional, national, seasonal
-ment	condition of	argument, endorsement, treatment, punishment
-ize	become	modernize, humanize, socialize, nationalize
-less	without	ageless, endless, lawless, faceless, effortless
-ness	state of being	happiness, sadness, heaviness, rudeness
-ious, -ous	characterized by	nutritious, studious, poisonous, lecherous
-ship	position held	fellowship, friendship, ownership, internship

As derivational morphemes constitute a type of bound morphemes, inflectional morphemes also belong to the bound morpheme category. **Inflectional morphemes** are affixes that are added to a word to assign a specific grammatical property to that word. There are only eight of them in English and they are all suffixes (see Table 4.3). Inflectional morphemes have the following properties that differentiate them from derivational morphemes:

a) Do not change the part of speech and/or the meaning of a word (e.g., *-er* in *bigger*).
b) Are required by syntax (e.g., The third person singular *-s* in *The boy likes to read*).
c) Typically occur with all members of some large class of morphemes (e.g., The plural *-s* in English).
d) Occur at the margin of a word.

Table 4.3 Inflectional Suffixes in English

Inflectional Suffix	Examples
Nouns:	
plural -s	the songs
possessive-'s	Mary's song
Verbs:	
3rd person singular -s	She writes beautifully.
progressive -ing	She is writing.
past tense -ed	She cooked.
past participle -en/-ed	She has eaten/worked.
Adjectives:	
comparative -er	smaller, bigger, quicker, closer
superlative -est	smallest, biggest, quickest, closest

4.4 Allomorphs

In Chapter 3, we explored the concept of allophones, predictable phonetic real-izations of a phoneme. Here, we consider **allomorphs**, the alternate phonetic forms of a morpheme. The plural morpheme -*s* in English, for example, has three allomorphs. In forming plural nouns, English speakers typically think about adding the plural morpheme -*s* at the end of nouns. However, the mor-pheme -*s* is uttered differently depending on the phonetic environment. Let us consider the following data:

[s]	[z]	[ɪz]
lips [lɪps]	trees [triz]	latches [lætʃɪz]
rocks [raks]	gums [gʌmz]	wretches [rɛtʃɪz]
bats [bæts]	twos [tuz]	fudges [fʌdʒɪz]
cats [kæts]	bells [bɛlz]	breezes [brizɪz]

As we learned in Chapter 3, we can list the phonetic environments of the three forms in question as follows:

[s]	[z]	[ɪz]
p—#	i—#	tʃ—#
k—#	m—#	tʃ—#
t—#	u—#	dʒ—#
t—#	l—#	z—#

(Note: "#" means word boundary.)

When we look at the sounds that are immediately to the left of [s], we notice that they are all voiceless sounds. In contrast, the sounds that occur immediately before [z] are all voiced sounds. The sounds that are immediately left of [ɪz] form a natural class, a special class of consonants called "sibilants". Sibilants are acoustically intense sounds produced by directing a stream of air with the tongue towards the sharp edge of the teeth, which are held close together. The sounds, [s], [z], [ʃ], [ʒ], [tʃ], and [dʒ], are sibilants in English.

To understand why [ɪz] is required for words that end in a sibilant, try attaching [s] to the end of *kiss* [kɪs] and [z] to the end of *hose* [hoʊz]. When we do that, we realize that it is difficult to say [kɪss] or [hoʊzz] with two [s]'s or [z]'s produced in quick succession and that the listener may not perceive that plural nouns were in fact meant by the speaker. However, by attaching [ɪz] at the end of these words, we can more easily communicate to the listener that they are plural.

Based on the data, we can write a phonological rule regarding the distribution of [s], [z], and [ɪz] as follows:

The English plural morpheme -*s* is pronounced as [s] following a noun that ends in a voiceless sound, as [z] following a noun that ends in a voiced sound, and as [ɪz] after a sibilant.

Likewise, the English past tense morpheme -*ed* has three allomorphs, [d], [t], and [ɪd], that work in similar ways. Consider the following data:

[t]	[d]	[ɪd]
sipped [sɪpt]	beamed [bimd]	ended [ɛndɪd]
dunked [dʌŋkt]	played [plɛɪd]	bunted [bʌntɪd]
cashed [kæʃt]	wintered [wɪntərd]	handed [hændɪd]
practiced [præktɪst]	logged [lagd]	hinted [hɪntɪd]

We can list the distribution of the three allomorphs as follows:

[t]	[d]	[ɪd]
p—#	m—#	d—#
k—#	ɪ—#	t—#
ʃ—#	r—#	d—#
s—#	g—#	t—#

Based on this list, the phonological distribution of [t], [d], and [ɪd] can be stated as follows:

The English past tense morpheme -*ed* is pronounced as [t] following a verb that ends in a voiceless sound, as [d] following a verb that ends in a voiced sound, and as [ɪd] after a verb that ends in either [t] or [d].

Yet another example of allomorphs in English involves the phonetic variants *a* and *an* for the indefinite article *a*. Here again, the use of one or the other form is determined by the phonetic environment—*a* is used before a word that begins with a consonant sound and *an* is used before a word that begins with a vowel sound (e.g., *a boat, a cat* vs. *an apple, an orange*). Inserting [n] between two vowels in *an apple* [ənæpl] and *an orange* [ənorɪndʒ] helps speakers avoid producing two vowels in succession and clearly communicates to the listener that a single item was meant in the utterance.

Voices From the Classroom 4.1—Teaching the Third Person Singular Morpheme -s

Sean Stinson, an elementary school ESOL teacher, asks his students to write a text on what they do on New Year's. A student might write, *I celebrate New Year's Day with my family and relatives.* Another student might write, *I make New Year's resolutions on New Year's Day.* The students then switch papers with a partner and rewrite their partner's text in the third person. So, the above sentences will be rewritten as, *Mariajose celebrates New Year's Day with her family and relatives* and *Yuanli makes New Year's resolutions on New Year's Day.* Students then get in small groups to orally summarize their partner's text in the third person. This helps students to listen for the third person singular morpheme and produce it correctly.

4.5 Inflection

Inflection is a morphological process that changes the form of a word to express a grammatical function or attribute. In the last section, we saw how the plural -s and the past tense -ed morphemes are attached to words in English to express **number** and **tense**. Inflection is commonly used in many languages of the world and can affect words that belong to various parts of speech.

In Spanish, different verb endings mark the grammatical concept of **person**. For example, the verb *hablar* ("to speak") can be conjugated in the present indicative as follows:

Yo hablo	"I speak"
Tú hablas	"You (singular, informal) speak"
Él/Ella/Usted habla	"He/She speaks", "You (singular, formal) speak"
Nosotros hablamos	"We speak"
Vosotros habláis	"You speak"
Ellos/Ellas/Ustedes hablan	"They/You (plural, formal) speak"

As can be seen in these examples, the verb endings communicate information about the person doing the action. And because the verb endings indicate who the subject of the sentence is, the subject can be dropped in Spanish without causing miscommunication. Thus, if someone were to say, *Hablamos español* without the first-person plural subject *nosotros* ("we"), we can conclude that the subject is *nosotros* from looking at the verb ending. For this reason, Spanish (along with a considerable number of the world's languages including Arabic, Chinese, Hungarian, Persian, and Polish) is considered a **null-subject language**, a language whose grammar permits an independent clause to lack an explicit subject (see Chapter 5 for more information).

For a language like English with very little inflection, however, omitting the subject is not allowed because the verb is not inflected according to the subject of the sentence. In fact, in English, the subject is required even in cases where a sentence has no **referent** at all (a referent is a person or thing to which a linguistic expression refers). For example, *Rains* is not an acceptable sentence in English. A dummy pronoun *it* must be added to produce a grammatically correct sentence, *It rains*. In most Romance languages, however, *Rains* is a perfectly fine sentence. Therefore, one can say, *Llueve* (Spanish), *Piove* (Italian), and *Chove* (Portuguese) in these null-subject languages.

Taking another example from Spanish, we can see that the grammatical concepts of **gender** and number are marked by different endings to nouns, adjectives, and determiners. In the following phrases, the *-o* ending signifies male while the *-a* ending signifies female. The *-s* morpheme is attached to the margin of the word to denote plurality. Notice that gender and number are marked not only in the noun (*niños, niñas*), but also in the determiner (*los, las*) and the adjective (*rubios, rubias*).

el	niño	rubio	"the blond boy"
la	niña	rubia	"the blond girl"
los	niños	rubios	"the blond boys"
las	niñas	rubias	"the blond girls"

Having determiner, noun, and adjective all agree in number and gender is a grammatical requirement in Spanish. However, English speakers often make errors in number and gender agreement in Spanish because (1) English does not have grammatical gender, and (2) it pluralizes nouns, but not the accompanying articles or adjectives. To help Spanish learners produce grammatical sentences then, teachers should explain these differences between the two languages explicitly and include exercises that help increase students' sensitivity to these features.

It is important for teachers to understand that different languages mark the same grammatical concepts quite differently. While plurality is expressed in Spanish (and in English) through the plural suffix *-s*, an overt affix is not required for expressing singularity. However, some languages inflect both singular and plural nouns. In Luganda, one of the major languages spoken in Uganda, both singular and plural nouns are marked with different prefixes. In the following data from Luganda, notice that the singular morpheme *omu-* marks a noun as singular while the plural morpheme *aba-* marks a noun as plural.

omusajja	"man"	abasajja	"men"
omukazi	"woman"	abakazi	"women"
omusawo	"doctor"	abasawo	"doctors"
omusika	"heir"	abasika	"heirs"
omulenzi	"boy"	abalenzi	"boys"

Another interesting difference in grammatical marking can be found when we compare Finnish to English. In Finnish, nouns are inflected to indicate meanings typically expressed by prepositions such as *in, to,* and *from* in English.

talo	"house" (subject)	talolla	"on the house"
talon	"house" (object)	talolta	"from the house"
talossa	"in the house"	talolle	"to the house"
talosta	"out of the house"	taloa	"part of the house"
taloon	"into the house"	talotta	"without the house"

Thus, a single inflected noun in Finnish (*talossa*) is equivalent to an entire prepositional phrase ("in the house") in English. This example shows that what constitutes a "word" or a "phrase" is not the same in all languages, but rather fluid from one language to another. Understanding cross-linguistic differences like this is important for teachers who are trying to help students gain mastery of second language features.

4.6 Other Morphological Processes

In addition to inflection, different languages use a variety of other morphological processes to form new words. These include compounding, reduplication, internal modification, and suppletion. In the following, we explain each of these with examples.

Compounding is the process of building a new word by combining two or more existing words. The component words of a compound may be of the same part of speech (e.g., *bookshelf*, composed of two nouns *book* and *shelf*; *bitter-sweet*, composed of two adjectives, *bitter* and *sweet*), or may belong to different parts of speech (e.g., *carsick*, composed of the noun *car* and the adjective *sick*; *someday*, composed of the determiner *some* and the noun *day*). In most compound words, the rightmost morpheme determines the part of the speech of the entire word. Thus, *whiteboard* is a noun because *board* is a noun, *babysit* is a verb because *sit* is a verb, and *statewide* is an adjective just as *wide* is.

Compound words in English are not represented consistently in writing. Some compound words are written as single words (*online, backbone, blackmail*), some with a hyphen (*sugar-free, off-campus, bone-dry*), and some as separate words (*on campus, school bus, decision making*). Regardless of how they are written, we can make some generalizations about how compound words are pronounced. For example, adjective-noun compound words in English have the primary stress falling on the first component of the compound (see Table 4.4). On the other hand, non-compound expressions involving an adjective and a noun typically have the primary stress falling on the second component.

Although the rules for forming compounds differ from language to language, compounding is a morphological process that is very common in many of the world's languages. For one, compounding helps languages to avoid creating brand new words and get more use out of existing words to express ideas. For example, in Korean, the word *karak* "strand" is attached to words that refer to various body parts to produce *bal<u>karak</u>* "toe", *son<u>karak</u>* "finger", and *mʌri<u>karak</u>* "hair". The words *bal*, *son*, and *mʌri* mean "foot", "hand", and "head" respectively. Thus, in Korean, toe literally means "foot strand" and finger, "hand strand", and hair, "head strand".

Compounding can also stretch the uses of whole classes of words by changing the part of speech. In Hindi, for example, a general verb *karnaa* ("to do") can be combined with many adjectives and nouns, to form verbs. Thus, *saaf karnaa*, which is a combination of the adjective *saaf* "clean" and *karnaa* "to do" means "to clean". *Nishchit karnaa*, a combination of the adjective *nishchit* "fixed" and *karnaa* "to do" means "to decide". The verb *karnaa* can also be attached to nouns such as *pyaar* ("love") and *mazaak* ("jest") to mean "to love" (*pyaar karnaa*) and "to joke" (*mazaak karnaa*).

While compounding is commonly used in many languages, some languages are more prone to forming new words through this process than others. English speakers who glimpse texts written in German often get the impression that words are generally longer in German than in English. This is because German allows for the combination of words that typically stay separate in English. Words like *krankenhausverzeichnis* "hospital directory", *behandlungsmethoden* "treatment methods", *massenaufstand* "mass uprising", and *familienmitgliedern* "family members" are compound nouns, whose meanings can be expressed with separate words in English. Likewise, *tischtennisball "ping pong ball"* is an amalgamation of three words, *tisch* "table", *tennis* "tennis", and *ball* "ball".

Table 4.4 Different Stress Placements in Compounds vs. Non-compounds

Compound	Non-Compound
bluébird "a type of American songbird"	*blue bírd* "any bird that has blue feathers"
whíteboard "a wipeable board"	*white boárd* "any board that is white"
strónghold "a place that has been fortified"	*strong hóld* "a grip that is powerful"

Understanding the German propensity to form new words in this way is useful for second language learners of German and can help them parse newly encountered words into smaller, more manageable chunks, rather than simply treat them as long, difficult words. The job of the German language teacher, then, is to demystify the principles of word formation in German so that they can help students in vocabulary acquisition.

Aside from compounding, another strategy that many languages use to form new words is reduplication. **Reduplication** is a morphological process that changes a word's meaning by repeating or copying all or part of the word. In Malay, duplication of root words can serve the same function that bound morphemes serve in other languages. For example, some nouns can be reduplicated to denote plurality. Examples include *buku-buku* "books", *pokok-pokok* "trees", and *orang-orang* "people", which are derived from *buku* "book", *pokok* "tree", and *orang* "person".

Some adjectives in Malay become adverbs when duplicated. Examples include *lambat-lambat* "slowly", *dalam-dalam*, "deeply" and *tajam-tajam* "sharply", derived from *lambat* "slow", *dalam* "deep", and *tajam* "sharp". In addition, some Malay verbs become nouns when partially reduplicated. For example, *sedu-seduan* "sobbing" is derived from *sedu* "to sob" and *tindak-tanduk* "action", from *tindak* "to act on". Partial reduplication also occurs in certain bound morphemes in Malay such as *haru-biru* "in great confusion", *dolak-dalik* "going back and forth", and *mundar-mandir* "walk aimlessly".

In English, we can find examples of full reduplication in words like *bye-bye*, *night-night*, and *no-no*. English also has partial reduplication in rhyming compounds such as, *walkie-talkie, mumbo-jumbo, itsy-bitsy, super-duper, hocus-pocus*, and *razzle-dazzle*, where the first word is reduplicated except for the onset of the first syllable.

Internal modification is a morphological process that substitutes one sound for another to mark a grammatical contrast. In English, internal modification can be observed in the formation of the past participle (e.g., *see/saw, steal/stole, make/made, ring/rang*). It can also be seen in the irregular plural forms of nouns (e.g., *man/men, woman/women, foot/feet, tooth/teeth, mouse/mice*). An internal modification can also involve suprasegmental features such as pitch and stress. Thus, some nouns become verbs by a change in the placement of stress (e.g., *réfund/refúnd, cónflict/conflíct, ínsult/insúlt*).

A whole set of English words can be learned by mastering this stress placement rule. Teachers can help students use the correct form of these words by presenting sentences such as, *Some people will go to great lengths to avoid _____ (cónflict). These results _____ (conflíct) with earlier findings.* Students can work in pairs to fill in the blanks and practice reading the sentences out loud to their partners, making sure to place stress accurately.

Related to these noun/verb pairs are another set of words like *decide/decisive, invade/invasive*, and *offend/offensive*, where a verb becomes an adjective when the ending sound *d* is replaced with *-sive*. When students are made aware of this principle of word formation, they can learn a whole new set of words relatively easily. There are also regularities in stress placement involving English words with suffixes *-y* and *-ic* such as *ecónomy/económic, demócracy/democrátic, geógraphy/geográphic,* and *philánthropy/philanthrópic.* Notice how the stressed vowel in a word with the suffix *-y* is reduced to a schwa when the word takes on the suffix *-ic.* Since many of these words are found in academic English, teachers' pointing out such patterns can facilitate students' vocabulary growth.

Finally, **suppletion** is a morphological process that marks a grammatical contrast by replacing a morpheme with a completely different morpheme. Suppletion involves related words that look nothing like each other. These are words that teachers often tell students to "just memorize". A good example of suppletion can be seen in English, where the pronoun *I* is used for the subject of the sentence and the pronoun *me* is used for the direct object of the sentence. There is similar contrast between *he* and *him, she* and *her, we* and *us,* and *they* and *them.* As can be seen in the following, **case** involves a change in a word's form to indicate its grammatical role in the sentence (as subject, direct object, and so on).

Nominative	Accusative	Possessive
I	me	my
he	him	his
she	her	her
we	us	our
they	them	their

Thus, nominative and accusative cases refer to the subject and direct object of the verb respectively, while possessive case refers to ownership. For each

---

Voices From the Classroom 4.2—Churchill's Trouble With Case

Winston Churchill, one of the greatest figures of the twentieth century, had considerable difficulty with Latin grammar as a schoolboy. The following is an excerpt from his autobiography, *My Early Life: 1874–1904.*

[The Form Master] produced a thin greeny-brown-covered book filled with words in different types of print.
"You have never done any Latin before, have you?" he said.
"No, sir."
"This is a Latin grammar." He opened it at a well-thumbed page. "You must learn this," he said, pointing to a number of words in a frame of lines. "I will come back in half an hour and see what you know."
Behold me then on a gloomy evening, with an aching heart, seated in front of the First Declension.

Mensa	a table
Mensa	o table
Mensam	a table
Mensae	of a table
Mensae	to or for a table
Mensa	by, with or from a table

What on earth did it mean? Where was the sense of it? It seemed absolute rigmarole to me. However, there was one thing I could always do: I could learn by heart. And I thereupon proceeded, as far as my private sorrows would allow, to memorise the acrostic-looking task which had been set me.

In due course the Master returned.

"Have you learnt it?" he asked.

"I think I can *say* it, sir", I replied; and I gabbled it off.

He seemed so satisfied with this that I was emboldened to ask a question.

"What does it mean, sir?"

"It means what it says. Mensa, a table. Mensa is a noun of the First Declension. There are five declensions. You have learnt the singular of the First Declension."

"But," I repeated, "what does it mean?"

"Mensa means a table," he answered.

"Then why does mensa also mean O table," I enquired, "and what does O table mean?"

"Mensa, O table, is the vocative case," he replied.

"But why O table?" I persisted in genuine curiosity.

"O table—you would use that in addressing a table, in invoking a table." And then seeing he was not carrying me with him, "You would use it in speaking to a table."

"But I never do," I blurted out in honest amazement.

"If you are impertinent, you will be punished, and punished, let me tell you, very severely," was his conclusive rejoinder.

Such was my first introduction to the classics from which, I have been told, many of our cleverest men have derived so much solace and profit.

From: Churchill, Winston. (1958). *My Early Life: 1874–1904*. New York: Simon & Schuster (pp. 10–12).

case, while the meaning of the word is related from column to column, the pronoun changes form completely.

Table 4.5 Suppletion in English Verbs

	Present	Past
Regular form	walk	walked
Regular form	chew	chewed
Suppletive form	go	went
Suppletive form	am	was

Table 4.6 Suppletion in English Adjectives

	Adjective	Comparative	Superlative
Regular form	big	bigger	biggest
Regular form	small	smaller	smallest
Suppletive form	good	better	best
Suppletive form	bad	worse	worst

Table 4.7 Suppletive Forms of the Adjectives "Good" and "Bad" in Some of the Romance Languages and Latin

	good	better/best	bad	worse/worst
French	bon	meilleur	mal	pire
Spanish	bueno	mejor	malo	peor
Italian	buono	migliore	male	peggiore
Catalan	bo	millor	mal	pitjor
Portuguese	bom	melhor	mau	pior
Latin	bonus	melior	malus	peior

In addition to the pronouns, the verbs *go* and *be* in English also have suppletive past tenses (see Table 4.5). Notice that there is simply no similarity between *go* and *went*, and between *am* and *was*. It is not possible to show a relationship between these words through a general rule because the forms involved in suppletion have different roots.

The same goes for English adjectives *good* and *bad*, which have suppletive comparative and superlative forms (Table 4.6).

The comparative and superlative of the adjective *good* and *bad* are also suppletive in the Romance languages, which have evolved from Latin (see Table 4.7). Notice the striking similarities among the five languages, whose connection to the original suppletive forms in Latin is easy to observe.

4.7 Teaching Principles of Word Formation to Students

How can knowledge of word formation help language learners? One of the most important tasks facing the language teacher is helping students learn new words and use them accurately in different contexts. Teachers can use a variety of strategies to help students in this regard.

For one, bilingual Spanish-English speakers can be taught to use related morphological structures in Spanish and English to understand sophisticated English lexical items and to expand their English vocabularies. Teachers can point out that a Spanish noun that ends in *-idad* almost always has an English cognate that ends in *-ity* (*actividad/activity, electricidad/electricity, velocidad/velocity*). Similarly, the Spanish bound morpheme *-mente* works very much like the English suffix *-ly* and changes an adjective to an adverb (*rápidamente/rapidly, perfectamente/perfectly, totalmente/totally*). If students already know the Spanish word, its equivalent in English can be pointed out. If they do not

---

Voices From the Classroom 4.3—"Superlatives Olympics"

Morphology definitely comes into play when I teach the grammar of comparatives and superlatives. After a lesson on how *-er* and *-est* endings change the meaning of adjectives, as well as an explanation of when to use *more, most, better*, and *best*, we have a Superlatives Olympics. Three teams send up one teammate for each event, and we compete to find out who can jump the highest, who has the longest hair, who can yell the loudest, who has the biggest feet, who has the smallest hands, who can write the fastest, who is the best singer, who is the coolest dancer, etc. Students get very competitive, and they use comparatives and superlatives to emphatically argue their teammates' victories (*Abdullah is not taller than Omar! Just look! Abdullah is shorter! Omar is the tallest!*)

Erica Ashton, ESL Teacher

---

know the word in either language, the Spanish and English words can be taught together to promote development of literacy in both languages.

Students can also benefit from having cognates pointed out and learning how to distinguish cognates from false cognates. **Cognates** are words that have the same linguistic derivation from the same original word or root. Examples of Spanish-English cognates include: *centro/center, colonia/colony, grupo/group, operación/operation, problema/problem, votar/vote*. Teachers can increase students' awareness of cognates by having students sort words in pairs. Teachers can give to each pair of students a set of word cards, each with either a word in Spanish or in English. The students sort and match the cognates (a card with the word *centro* would be matched with a card with word *center*, *grupo* would be matched with *group*, and so on). Students then discuss in pairs what the matched words have in common. Students can talk about similarities in the sounds between the cognates and what strategies they might use to spell the words correctly in both languages.

Cognates appear across many Indo-European languages. As can be seen in Table 4.8, many science- and technology-related words are cognates that share common Greek and Latin roots such as *aud, eco, meta, morph*, and *organ*.

When teaching correspondences between cognates found in different languages, it is important to help students distinguish true cognates from false cognates. **False cognates** are pairs of words that appear to be cognates because of similar sounds (and meaning) but in fact are not cognates because they have different origins. Examples of false Spanish-English cognates include: *sano/ sane* (*sano* means *healthy*), *embarazada/embarrassed* (*embarazada* means *pregnant*), *la noticia/notice* (*noticia* means *news*), *la librería/library* (*librería* means *bookstore*), *el negocio/negotiation* (*negocio* means *business*), *el suceso/ success* (*suceso* means *event*), *el éxito/exit* (*éxito* means *success*). To help students identify false cognates, teachers can have them work in pairs to find as many false cognates as they can from a given list of words. Students can talk about similarities in the appearance and sounds of false cognates and the true meaning of the words. Each group of students can then share a pair of false

---

Voices From the Classroom 4.4—Cognates Have to be Explicitly Taught, Not Assumed

I was surprised when cognates were not as readily apparent to my Spanish-speaking students as I anticipated that they would be. That said, upon reflection on my own experience learning German, I could see the same effects were present when I was attempting to learn German words and phrases that I now can recognize as being very similar in construction and meaning, but different in pronunciation (e.g., *hunde* vs. *hound, freunde* vs. *friend, wasser* vs. *water*). The ability to relate form, meaning, and sounds is important for learning new words and shows how language learning is multi-modal/multi-sensory. Here, teachers can help students see connections that may not be readily apparent to them.

Steve Wagoner, Adult ESL Teacher

---

cognates they found with the whole class.

When teaching vocabulary, it is important for teachers to understand that knowing a word requires not only knowing its meaning, but also knowing how it relates to similar forms. For example, the word *nutrient* is related to words

Table 4.8 Science Cognates in Select Languages

English	Spanish	Italian	French	German
audiology	audiología	audiologia	audiologie	audiologie
ecology	ecología	ecologia	écologie	ökologie
metamorphosis	metamorfosis	metamorfosi	métamorphosse	metamorphose
organism	organismo	organismo	organisme	organismus

with different affixes such as *nutrition, nutritious, nutritionist,* and *nutritional.* Knowing how each form can be used accurately within a sentence is as important as knowing the meanings of the individual words. Thus, students can say, "The foods you eat supply your body with the <u>nutrients</u> you need" but not "Poor <u>nutrients</u> may increase your risk of heart disease and diabetes". Teachers can explain why the word *nutrition* is a more accurate term in the second sentence by drawing students' attention to the small but important difference in the meanings of these closely related words (*nutrient* meaning the substance that provides nourishment for maintaining a healthy body, as opposed to *nutrition,* which means the process of providing nourishment).

Knowing a word also means understanding how it relates to other related words and concepts (e.g., *calories, carbohydrates, fats, proteins, vitamins, minerals*). New words are more meaningful when they are understood in conjunction with other words related to the same general topic. The good news for language teachers is that students are already exposed to these and many academic words in everyday conversations and in their encounters with a variety of written materials available on- and off-line. Since students learn vocabulary most effectively in real context and related to topics that interest them, teachers should expose students to reading materials that they care about and encourage them to read widely. In all of this, teachers should remember that helping students to gain a deeper understanding of individual words and how to use them accurately is as important as helping them to acquire more vocabulary.

Recommended Websites

¡Colorín Colorado! offers a wealth of bilingual, research-based information, activities, and advice for educators and families of English language learners. www.colorincolorado.org/
WordSpy is an online bank of new words added to the English language. www.wordspy.com/

Further Reading

Arnoff, M., & Fudeman, K. (2010). *What is morphology?* (2nd ed.). Malden, MA: Wiley-Blackwell.

Haspelmath, M., & Sims, A. (2010). *Understanding morphology* (2nd ed.). New York: Oxford University Press.

Katamba, F., & Stonham, J. (2006). *Morphology* (2nd ed.). London: Palgrave Macmillan.

Stahl, S. A., & Nagy, W. E. (2006). *Teaching word meanings*. Mahwah, NJ: Erlbaum.

Exercises

1. Consider the following words in English. For each word, determine whether it is a simple word (made up of a single morpheme) or a complex word (composed of two or more morphemes). For the complex words you identified, circle all the bound morphemes.

(a) bike	(e) greener	(i) friendship	(m) habitual
(b) clever	(f) review	(j) gladness	(n) nonbinding
(c) lightly	(g) distrust	(k) forest	(o) active
(d) respectful	(h) yellowish	(l) uncaring	(p) statement

2. The following words are made up of two or more morphemes. For each word, isolate the morphemes and determine whether each morpheme is free or bound. For each bound morpheme, determine if it is derivational or inflectional.

(a) joyful	(e) unhealthy	(i) multicultural	(m) globalization
(b) staplers	(f) boyfriend	(j) crazier	(n) thunderstorm
(c) glorify	(g) judgment	(k) recreational	(o) tallest
(d) birthdays	(h) unthinkable	(l) colorlessness	(p) governments

3. Consider the two columns of words below and answer the questions that follow.

straight	straighten
hard	harden
sweet	sweeten
awake	awaken
ripe	ripen
bright	brighten
worse	worsen

   a) What part of speech does the suffix -*en* attach to?

   b) What part of speech is the resulting word after the suffix -*en* has been attached?

   c) How does the suffix -*en* change the meaning of the word that it is attached to?

4. Each word in the following two lists is preceded by a prefix *un-*.

undo	unafraid
unbend	unconscious
unfold	unfair
unpack	unable
unwind	unlucky
unzip	uncertain
untangle	unseen

a) What part of speech are the words in the left column before and after the prefix *un-* is attached? What part of speech are the words in the right column before and after the prefix *un-* is attached?

b) How does the prefix *un-* change the meaning of the word it attaches to in the left column? How does the prefix *un-* change the meaning of the word it attaches to in the right column? How is the change of meaning in the left column different from that in the right column?

c) Based on this evidence, would you say that the two columns represent words with two different prefixes?

5. The Turkish plural suffix has two allomorphs, *-lar* and *-ler*. Consider the following data from Turkish and determine the phonetic environments in which each allomorph is used. Note that "ü" is a high front rounded vowel, "ö", a mid front rounded vowel, and "ı", a high back unrounded vowel. (Hint: Rather than simply list the sound that is immediately to the left of the allomorph, try looking at the last vowel in the root word. See if you can identify any natural class among the last vowels in the left column vs. the last vowels in the right column.)

-lar		*-ler*	
kitap "book"	kitaplar "books"	ev "house"	evler "houses"
araba "car"	arabalar "cars"	gün "day"	günler "days"
yol "way"	yollar "ways"	göz "eye"	gözler "eyes"
okul "school"	okullar "schools"	el "hand"	eller "hands"
kız "girl"	kızlar "girls"	diz "knee"	dizler "knees"

6. Working with a partner, select a paragraph in any news article and list as many compounds as you can find. Remember that compounds can be a noun (*football, distance learning, standby*), a verb (*freeze-dry, highlight, blackmail*), an adjective (*awe-inspiring, blue-green, over-ripe*), an adverb (*forthwith, straightaway*), or a preposition (*within, without*), and can be written as single words, with a hyphen, or as separate words.

5 Syntax

The Analysis of Sentences

5.1 Introduction

Syntax is the study of sentence structure. Every language has rules that govern how the words in that language come together to form phrases, clauses, and sentences. This is the layer of language that informs us that while some orders work just fine (*why did he eat the sandwich?*) others do not work at all (*he eat the sandwich did why?*). It is important to note that while there are differences in these rules from language to language, all languages have their own sets of rules. Dialects and creoles have systematic rules as well.

What does it mean for languages to have rules for sentence structure? It means that words cannot be combined randomly. For instance, suppose you give someone a stack of eight index cards with a different word on each card. The cards have the following words written on them: *all, comedian, funny, of, laugh, made, the, us*. Theoretically, there are 40,320 possible combinations. However, if you give this stack of cards to a large group of English speakers and ask them to create a sentence using all the cards, they will all likely come up with the same sentence (that's .002% of all the possible combinations). The fact that they can do that suggests that word combinations in language are not random.

This chapter shows how words are grouped into syntactic categories, and how sentences have a hierarchical design in which words are gathered into successively larger structural units. You will learn how to diagram phrase structure trees, and derive questions from statements as well as passive sentences from active sentences. This chapter will show how to focus learners' attention on grammatical form by providing tasks that require the use of certain structures (i.e., implicit teaching of grammar). It will also provide strategies for helping learners navigate dense academic texts with complex sentences.

5.2 Constituency

Often, we think of phrases, clauses, and sentences as being a string of words. Certainly, when we hear a sentence or produce an utterance, it comes out in a continuous string. However, linguists have identified that there are groupings in sentences that form a hierarchy. Words come together to form phrases, and these phrases come together to form clauses. This idea that words are grouped into units is called **constituency**. Let us consider the following examples.

(1) They quickly ran out the door.
(2) They quickly found out the truth.

On the surface, the two preceding sentences look quite similar in structure. Both sentences have the same subject *they*, both sentences have an adverb, verb, and an *out the* construction to end the sentence. In fact, the sentences are identical on the surface except for two words. However, the sentences are structurally quite different. One way to explore that is by moving some parts of the sentence around. Let us invert the first sentence:

(3) Out the door, they quickly ran.

When you invert the first sentence, it sounds fine, rather like a construction you would see in a children's book. But what happens when you invert (2)?

(4) *Out the truth, they quickly found.

The result is ungrammaticality (notated with an asterisk). Even though two sentences may appear similar on the surface, the internal structure reveals otherwise. This tells us that *out the door* in (1) is a constituent because it can be moved as a unit, but *out the truth* in (2) is not a constituent because it cannot be moved.[1] If sentences were a string of words with no hierarchy, we should be able to apply the same test to both and have the same outcome. In fact, we should be able to group words any which way. However, tests of constituency show that there are natural groupings of words that form a unit that prevent some of these tests, like movement.

  Constituents can be individual words, phrases, and clauses. Although every language has different rules, there are some tests of constituency that work across many of the world's languages. We have already seen the movement test. Another test is substitution. The idea is that if a grouping of words forms a constituent, then it should be substitutable. Let us explore this further with another example.

(5) A woman from the cafe found my backpack.

In this example, there are a number of constituents that can be identified. Every word by itself is a constituent, of course, but there are several phrases embedded within. Since phrases are constituents, it follows that phrases can be substitutable. In English, one good way to identify a noun phrase is to see if it can be substituted with a pronoun, because pronouns are stand-ins for noun phrases. Let's suppose we suspect that *a woman* is a noun phrase. If so, it should be substitutable with the pronoun *she*.

(6) *<u>She</u> from the cafe found my backpack.

Does the test work? No, it sounds quite bad to substitute *a woman* with *she* in this sentence. That tells us that *a woman* by itself is not a noun phrase. However, if we extend the test and substitute *a woman from the cafe* with the pronoun, we have a much better result. This tells us that *a woman from the cafe* is a noun phrase and therefore a constituent.

(7) <u>She</u> found my backpack.

Both the movement and the substitution tests are helpful in identifying constituents. It is important to recognize where constituents are because they are vital in building phrases from words, and clauses from phrases, as we will see next.

5.3 Parts of Speech

To start, let us talk about **parts of speech**. Different words have different grammatical functions. We are often taught in school that nouns are people, places, or things, and verbs are actions. However, sometimes those definitions lead us to the wrong conclusion. Consider (8) below.

(8) *baby*

    a.   The baby cried.
    b.   My parents baby me.
    c.   I knit a baby blanket.

If we look at the word *baby* in isolation, we would quickly evaluate that the word is a noun because it is a person. However, instead of relying only on meaning, if you look at both the morphological clues and where it occurs in the sentence (a clue we call *distribution*), you will realize that the word *baby* functions differently in each example in (8). In (8a) the word *baby* can be pluralized to *babies* and comes after the article *the*, so it is a noun. In (8b) the word *baby* can be changed to past tense *babied* and comes after the subject of the sentence, so it is a verb. In (8c) the word *baby* comes before a noun and after an article, and it can be substituted for a different descriptor like *soft*, so it is an adjective. These rules and tests are specific to English, but every language has rules and tests that are specific to that language that can be utilized.

The basic nine parts of speech that we will cover in this chapter are nouns (N), verbs (V), adjectives (A), adverbs (Adv), prepositions (P), determiners (D), auxiliaries (Aux), complementizers (C), and conjunctions (Conj). The parts of speech and characteristics of each one for English can be found in Table 5.1.

Nouns are open class words that generally refer to people, places, events, things, and ideas. As discussed in Chapter 4, open classes are parts of speech where new words enter the category frequently. Nouns can be proper nouns or common nouns. Proper nouns are ones that refer to a specific person, place, event, thing, or idea, such as *George, Wisconsin, Labor Day, The Statue of Liberty*. However, the most typical noun is a common noun, and these nouns are the ones that tend to obey the characteristics listed in Table 5.1: they can

Table 5.1 Parts of Speech and Their Characteristics

Part of Speech	Characteristics	Examples in context
Noun (N)	can form a plural can take a possessive can occur after determiners	The <u>song</u> was beautiful. <u>Melissa</u> asked me to bring the keys. We found no <u>evidence</u> for the theory.
Verb (V)	can take past tense can take *-ing* ending can take *-ed/-en* participle ending occurs after auxiliaries like *should, has, does*	He is <u>studying</u> biology. Our group will <u>present</u> first. Dr. Lau had <u>prepared</u> a speech. They <u>caught</u> a huge insect.
Adjective (A)	can take comparative forms (*-er, more X*) can take superlative forms (*-est, most X*) can occur before a noun can occur in sentences with the verb *to be* (e.g. She is *tall*) can be modified by an adverb	The <u>sweet</u> baby cooed happily. Those desserts are very <u>decadent</u>. My sister is <u>taller</u> than me.
Adverb (Adv)	can take *-ly* ending (not always a guarantee) can be modified by *very* or *too* can modify verbs, adjectives, prepositions, or other adverbs	Jorge <u>regretfully</u> cannot come. Not too <u>surprisingly</u>, there were many leftovers. The package was delivered <u>fast</u>.
Auxiliary (Aux)	comes before a verb can have more than one	She <u>has</u> seen the movie ten times. I <u>might have</u> opened it early. They <u>were</u> not eating yet.
Preposition (P)	occur before noun phrases cannot be inflected	Leave the homework <u>on</u> the desk. Hester lived <u>across</u> the street. The numbers <u>in</u> the table don't add up.
Determiner (D)	cannot be inflected can come before a noun cannot have more than one determiner in a noun phrase (*the my dog Rex)	<u>My</u> headache is better now. We found <u>these</u> papers in the file. Lia messaged us about <u>the</u> meeting.
Complementizer (C)	can begin a new clause cannot be inflected	They closed the school <u>because</u> of the snowstorm. <u>That</u> you won first place surprised no one. Please pick up a syllabus <u>if</u> you didn't get one.
Conjunctions (Conj)	cannot be inflected	My father <u>and</u> I share the same hobbies. Do they want the chicken <u>or</u> steak?

take a plural morpheme (*cake, cakes*), they can take possessives (*dog, dog's*), and they can come after determiners (*desert, the desert*). Common nouns can be further divided into two categories: count nouns and mass nouns. Count nouns are ones that can be counted with a numeral or a quantifier, and can be pluralized (e.g., *one shoe, two shoes, many shoes; one idea, two ideas, many ideas; one person, two people, many people*). Mass nouns, however, are ones that usually refer to a group, a substance, or a whole. Mass nouns typically cannot be counted with a numeral or quantifier, and they sound awkward when pluralized (e.g., *one furniture, *two furnitures, *many furnitures).

Verbs are one of the more complex parts of speech in language. Verbs in English only sometimes refer to actions, but are better characterized by their function: verbs drive the clause by functioning as the **predicate**. Verbs can take the past tense (*played, broke, ate*), can take progressive participle-*ing* ending (*playing, breaking, eating*), can take the past participle-*ed/-en* ending (*played, broken, eaten*), and can come after auxiliaries (*has played, will break, must have eaten*).

Adjectives are open class words whose one job is to modify nouns. They can modify nouns by preceding them (*funny joke, delicious meal*) or following a form of the verb *to be* (*the joke was funny, that meal is delicious*). Adjectives can take comparative forms (*funnier, more delicious*) and superlative forms (*funniest, most delicious*). Adjectives can also be modified by an adverb (*very funny joke, exceedingly delicious meal*).

Adverbs are open class modifiers too, but they do the job of modifying everything except nouns. Adverbs can modify verbs (*walk quickly*), adjectives (*very cold*), prepositions (*just across the street*), or even other adverbs (*too happily*). They are easiest to identify when they carry the -*ly* suffix, but this is not always a guarantee that the word is an adverb (*lovely*). Because adverbs modify so many of the other parts of speech, their position within a sentence can be very flexible.

Auxiliaries are words that precede verbs, and provide information such as conditionality, future expression, aspect, and mood. While some languages use verb endings to encode this information, English does this through auxiliaries that come before the verb. Auxiliaries can take the form of the verb *to be* (*was singing, are returned*), to have (*has finished, had informed*), and modals (*will go, should decide, can visit, might try*).

The remaining four parts of speech are all closed class words. The consequence of this is that there is a strict set of words that belong to the categories that cannot easily change. Furthermore, these words cannot be **inflected** with prefixes or suffixes. **Prepositions** are words that indicate relationships in space and time and are usually followed by a noun phrase (*in the dark, across the street, before class*). **Determiners** are words that precede nouns and provide information such as (in)definiteness (*the homework, a tree*), quantification (*some burgers, much water*), possession (*my house, their computer*), or demonstrative (*this research, those fish*). **Complementizers** are words that connect clauses together, usually in order to embed one into another (*she said that we could go, I was tired because I woke up early*). Finally, **conjunctions** are words that join two words, phrases, or clauses of equal weight (*he played the violin and recited a poem, do you want coffee or tea*).

5.4 Phrase Structure

Phrases are units of language (constituents) that are just above the level of words. Phrases can consist of a single word, as in (9), or many words, as in (10).

(9) <u>Ella</u> found my backpack.
(10) <u>The tall woman in the green sweatshirt from the cafe</u> found my backpack.

There are many kinds of phrases, but the main ones we will discuss in this book are the following: noun phrase (NP), verb phrase (VP), adjective phrase (AP), adverb phrase (AdvP), and prepositional phrase (PP). In Table 5.2, you can see some examples of each type of phrase. Phrases are generally written out with square brackets around them to show their boundaries.

The most simple kind of phrase has only one word in it. At the bare minimum, a phrase has to contain a head. The **head** of a phrase is the most important word, the word without which the phrase would be pointless, like a birthday party without the birthday person. The head is the VIP of the phrase. Thus, if you have a single-word phrase, that word is most assuredly the head of that phrase because a phrase has to have a head. For example, in the NP [*Sarah*], the head of the phrase is the noun *Sarah*. In a slightly longer NP [*these striped socks*], there still needs to be an N head, *socks*, but there are other words that make up the phrase. Without the head noun *socks*, the noun phrase would be rather meaningless. You might have noticed that the phrase (NP) and the head (N) match in type. The head of a VP is a V, the head of an AP is an A, and so on. That is the first main fact about heads and phrases:

Fact 1: The category of the head matches the category of the phrase.

If you look at the examples of phrases in Table 5.2, you will see that the underlined heads are of the same category (e.g., a noun is the head of the noun phrase). In short, the phrase and the head have to match. The two have a close relationship.

Another observation you might make when you look at the examples in Table 5.2 is that for every phrase, there is just one head underlined. This gives way to another fact about heads and phrases:

Fact 2: For every one phrase, there is one head.

The head and the phrase have an exclusive 1:1 relationship that cannot be broken.

You might have also noticed that within some of the phrases, there are other phrases within them. Indeed, phrases are often found within other phrases. Prepositional phrases, for example, often contain a noun phrase: the PP [*up the tree*] contains a P head, *up*, and the NP [*the tree*]. Prepositional phrases can also contain an adverb phrase just before the preposition, such as PP [*somewhat in the way*], where *somewhat* is the AdvP containing the adverb head *somewhat*. Often, linguists will use brackets to indicate where the phrase boundaries are: [$_{PP}$ [$_{AdvP}$ *somewhat*] *in* [$_{NP}$ *the way*]]. This notation shows that the PP contains the head P, of course, but also an AdvP and a NP. This brings us to our final fact about heads and phrases:

Fact 3: The head determines the selectional properties for the phrase.

In other words, the head decides what other elements can join a phrase and what cannot, like an exclusive clique. These rules are referred to as **phrase structure rules**, and every language has them. The phrase structure rules for English can be seen in Table 5.2. These rules are basically templates for each type of phrase. It gives you information about what constituents can be in the phrase, and it also tells you the position that the constituent can go. The elements that are in parentheses are optional. But beyond just being a formula, what is truly fascinating about phrase structure is that it is recursive; in other words, in an NP you might find a PP, and in that PP there is another NP, and in that NP there is yet another PP, and so on and so forth: *The girl in the photo of the class from the school on the corner of the street . . . .* There is theoretically no limit to how far you can go, other than the fact that most people will have forgotten what they were trying to say in the first place. This recursive nature of language is often cited as a feature of **generative grammar**, in that you can come up with an infinite number of utterances from a small subset of rules. It is infinitely generative.

Voices From the Classroom 5.1—Teaching Vocabulary Involves Not Only Reviewing the Meaning of the Word but Also Its Relationship to Other Words in the Sentence

It's useful to help students break down sentences into parts. I teach parts of speech and break sentences into chunks: subject, verb, and object, but I don't have students diagram sentences. I do not go too deep, but knowledge of how phrases are constructed is huge. Some verbs require direct objects. Native English speakers know this automatically, but ESL students need to be taught which verbs need a direct object and which need an indirect object. Sometimes a student says, *I give her.* A native English speaker knows it is wrong but may not be able to explain why it should be *I give it to her.* Teachers can show students which verbs need direct and indirect objects.

Hilary Reintges, Adult ESL Teacher

Table 5.2 Phrases in English

Phrase Type	Phrase Structure Rules	Examples (*head*)
Noun Phrase (NP)	NP → (D) (AP) N (PP)	*Sarah* A *teacher* These striped *socks* *House* on the corner of the street
Verb Phrase (VP)	VP → (AdvP) V (AdvP) (NP) (AdvP) (PP) (AdvP)	*Sleep* Really *sings* well *Practice* the drums Carefully *decide* on the verdict
Adjective Phrase (AP)	AP → (AdvP) A	*Heavy* Very *happy* Disgustingly *wealthy*
Adverb Phrase (AdvP)	AdvP → (AdvP) Adv	*Quickly* Extremely *delicately*
Prepositional Phrase (PP)	PP → (AdvP) P (NP)	*Off* *Up* the tree *With* my good friends Somewhat *in* the way

5.5 Drawing Tree Diagrams

A **tree diagram** is a typical way that linguists represent the inner workings of phrases and sentences. They are called trees because of the way different constituents branch off from other parts of the structure. These are often easier to read than the bracket notation we showed you in Table 5.2 because it visually represents the groupings in a dimensional rather than linear format. Tree diagrams show the relationship that words have to other words. They also demonstrate the hierarchy within phrases, clauses, and sentences.

Let us learn some basic terms for the parts of a tree diagram. Figure 5.1 presents an abstract tree for us to reference. Each joint of a tree is called a **node**; therefore, every letter on the tree in Figure 5.1 is a node. **Terminal nodes** are the ones at the ends of the branches, like B, D, E, G, and I. Also, **mother, daughter**, and **sister** are relationships between nodes. Mothers are nodes one level directly above the node in question. So for instance, C is the mother of D, E, and F. F is the mother of G and H. Daughters are the other way around, so D is the daughter of C, and C is the daughter of A. Sisters are ones that have a common mother, so B and C are sisters, and D, E, and F are sisters.

Recall that sentences are not just strings of words, but rather groupings called constituents. How we represent them on the tree is quite indicative of that property: to find a constituent on a tree diagram, identify a node and everything under it. Thus, C and all its daughters and granddaughters and great-granddaughters make up one constituent. H and I are constituents. D and E alone are NOT constituents together, because we have left out F and everything under it. Much like a family event, if you are inviting one sibling, you have to invite all the siblings.

Now, let us consider some good phrases and bad phrases. The good phrases in Figure 5.2 all obey the three main facts: the phrase and the head match in type, there is a 1:1 match between a phrase and its head, and the phrase only contains elements that are allowed for that phrase type. The bad phrases in Figure 5.3 break one or more of these rules. Tree 4 has two NPs and one VP, but they should then have two N heads and one V head. Also, NPs do not have VPs within them, per our phrase structure rule for NPs. In Tree 5, the head and the phrase do not match. And in Tree 6, the N head does not have a phrase.

Now let us draw some tree diagrams of our own, starting with a simple noun phrase, [*the book*]. The first step is to identify the parts of speech of all the

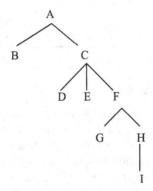

Figure 5.1 Sample Tree Diagram

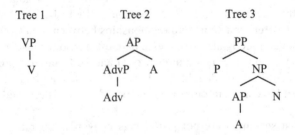

Figure 5.2 Good Phrase Structure Trees

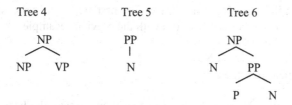

Figure 5.3 Bad Phrase Structure Trees

words in the phrase. A good way to do this is to write out the sentence and write the parts of speech above each word.

(11) D N

    the book

Next, we identify the head of the noun phrase. Recall that nouns must match in type to the phrase; in a noun phrase, the head must be a noun. Since there is only one noun in (11), identifying the head noun is quite simple: the head is *book*. The next step is to deal with the other words in the phrase. The only other word in this phrase is a determiner, but those are not one of the five phrases we are covering (NP, VP, PP, AP, AdvP).[2] Now, we are ready to diagram the NP [*the book*]. First we start with the NP at the top.

NP

Now, according to the NP phrase structure rule (NP → (D)(AP)N(PP)), we can have all kinds of elements branching off it. However, we only really have the D and the N in this case. Thus, we draw the determiner and noun branching off the NP.

NP
D   N

This tree diagram shows that the NP consists of a determiner and a noun, *the* and *book*. There are no other embedded phrases within it. This is a very basic tree, but it is quite common. We can now write the words under the terminal nodes to finish this tree diagram.

NP
D   N
the book

    Let us diagram another one that is slightly more complex. Consider the phrase [*a woman from the café*] which we saw earlier in the chapter. We have already identified it as a noun phrase. The first step is to write the parts of speech above each word like we did with the previous example.

(12) D N P D N
     a woman from the café

Next, we want to identify the head of the noun phrase. The head of a noun phrase must be a noun according to Fact 1, so that helps narrow down the choices. In this case, *woman* is the head of this noun phrase because it is the most important noun in the phrase.

    Now that we have found the head of the phrase, we turn our attention to the remaining words. Keeping in mind the five types of phrases we have learned about in this chapter (NP, VP, PP, AP, AdvP), identify any phrases you see within the entire noun phrase. Since we know that a head cannot exist without a phrase, a good place to start would be to see if there are any lone heads that do not yet have a phrase. The noun *café* does not have a noun phrase yet, and the preposition *from* does not have a prepositional phrase yet. [*The café*] forms an NP which is structurally exactly like [*the book*] from the previous example. Referencing the phrase structure rules in Table 5.2, a PP almost always has an NP in it. In fact, the PP [*from the café*] is made up of the head P *from* and the NP [*the café*]. Here is a bracketed version in (13).

(13) D N   P   D N
     [$_{NP}$ a woman [$_{PP}$ from [$_{NP}$ the café]]]

The brackets show us that within the large noun phrase, there is an embedded prepositional phrase, and within that prepositional phrase, there is another noun phrase.

    Having parsed the sentence, we are ready to draw the tree. To draw the tree top down, we start with the NP node:

NP

Then we have three daughter nodes branching off: D, N, and PP.

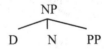

Next, from the PP node there are two nodes: P and NP.

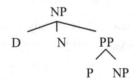

Finally, the NP node branches down into the components of the NP node.

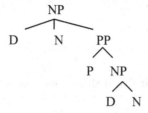

Then, we just fill in the terminal nodes with the words.

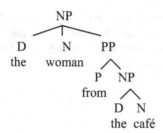

Once again, what we learn from this tree is that there are groupings within this phrase. There are phrases, and the head noun is modified by the elements that are sisters to it. Another important piece of information that we can derive from the tree is that everything that is a sister to the head is supporting or modifying the head in some way. The D *the* is giving information about *woman* (that she is a specific, definite, previously mentioned woman). The PP [*from the café*], a sister to the head, is modifying *woman* as well. In linear form, it may be difficult to see that relationship—that all signs point to the head noun *woman*—but in the tree diagram, it is much easier to see and identify the head and all of its modifiers. This is why linguists like such diagrams; trees allow us to analyze the structures more accurately and easily.

5.6 Clauses

Thus far, we have talked about words coming together to form phrases. The next level of syntax is the **clause**, which is made up of several phrases coming together. A clause is a constituent containing a **subject** and a predicate. Subjects are typically noun phrases. Predicates are typically verb phrases. The subject and the predicate come together to form the clause. Here is a simple example clause.

(14) They laughed.

In (14), the subject is NP [*they*] and the predicate is the VP [*laughed*]. The only new element in drawing tree diagrams for clauses is the S-node (where S stands for *sentence*), which connects the subject and the predicate.

(15)

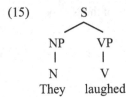

Let us try another example that is slightly more complex. Consider the clause in (16).

(16) My boss signed the papers.

In this example, the subject is the NP [*my boss*] and the predicate is the VP [*signed the papers*]. To diagram the sentence, we put the NP and VP together using the S-node. The rest of the tree, which includes drawing out NPs and VPs, is exactly what we have done earlier.

(17)

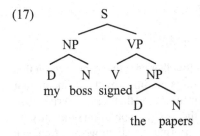

How do you identify the subject and the predicate? Earlier in the chapter we talked about a few tests for constituency like movement and substitution. Subjects in English are typically noun phrases, and we have learned that noun phrases can be substituted with a pronoun. Thus, to test whether something is a subject or not, try to substitute it with a pronoun. Let us take a look at the clauses in (18) and run the test on each one, as in (19).

(18) a. Tao sings really well.
      b. The birds found a nest.
      c. Mr. Sanders and I came to an agreement.
      d. The team from the leading school in the area won the championship.

(19) a. <u>He</u> sings really well.
      b. <u>They</u> found a nest.
      c. <u>We</u> came to an agreement.
      d. <u>It</u> won the championship. or <u>They</u> won the championship.

The substitution test with a pronoun reveals that *Tao, the birds, Mr. Sanders and I*, and *the team from the leading school in the area* are the subjects of these clauses.

You can also identify the subject by turning the sentence into a clarification question. A clarification question is an echo question with emphasis on the **wh-word** (such as *what* or *who*) that is used when you want someone to repeat what they just said. In this case, you can turn each into a clarification question, like in (20):

(20) a. <u>Who</u> sings really well?
    b. <u>Who</u> found a nest?
    c. <u>Who</u> came to an agreement?
    d. <u>Who</u> won the championship?

The answer to the questions will be your subject.

Predicates can be identified with a substitution test, too. Typically, English predicates can be substituted with *do so*. Let us run this substitution on our clauses from (18) in (21).

(21) a. Tao <u>does so</u>.
    b. The birds <u>did so</u>.
    c. Mr. Sanders and I <u>did so</u>.
    d. The team from the leading school in the area <u>did so</u>.

The *do so* substitution test reveals that *sings really well, found a nest, came to an agreement,* and *won the championship* are the predicates. It's important to remember that when you do the substitution test, you are not adding extra words or altering the remaining ones. Like a science experiment, we want to test one variable at a time. If you alter more than one thing at a time, you don't know whether the test actually worked, or some other element just made it look like it did.

Clauses come in two main varieties. The first type of clause is an **independent clause**. It is named such because it can stand alone, like the examples in (22). Independent clauses are sentences.

(22) a. Jill ran.
    b. The student studied.
    c. Every attendee received an award.
    d. The package was delivered to the wrong house.

The second type of clause is a **dependent clause,** or **embedded clause**. Dependent clauses usually begin with a complementizer, or a particle that serves as a connector to the main sentence, as in (23).

(23) a. Because Jill ran
    b. What the student studied
    c. That every attendee received an award
    d. If the package was delivered to the wrong house

Dependent clauses are usually found embedded within an independent clause.

(24)   a.   Jack dropped out of the race <u>because Jill ran</u>.
      b.   I don't know <u>what the student studied</u>.
      c.   <u>That every attendee received an award</u> surprised us all.
      d.   We'll see <u>if the package was delivered to the wrong house</u>.

In formal spoken English and in most written registers of English, dependent clauses typically cannot stand alone. However, it is important to note that it is not ungrammatical or wrong; it is simply a usage etiquette rule. It's not atypical to hear dependent clauses by themselves in spoken English or within informal registers of written English.

    Related to this, in formal written English, you may have heard of the terms **run-on** and **fragment**. Run-ons are two independent clauses in one sentence, which usually sounds like just that; two sentences fused together (*The student studied she got an A in her class*). To remedy a run-on, students can (a) separate them into two different sentences, (b) put a semicolon between the two clauses if the clauses are related, or (c) turn one of the sentences into a dependent clause by adding a complementizer. An example of each remedy can be seen in (25).

(25)   a.   The student studied. She got an A in her class.
      b.   The student studied; she got an A in her class.
      c.   <u>Because</u> the student studied, she got an A in her class.

A fragment, on the other hand, is a clause that is missing something. It could be an independent clause missing a subject (*found no relationship between the two variables*) or missing a predicate (*the researchers from the institute with*

Voices From the Classroom 5.2—Word Order in Embedded Questions

I like to use large word cards to help students grasp word order. For example, if we are learning about embedded questions, I will write out "where", "is", "the", "bathroom", and "?" on separate cards big enough for the whole class to see. I hand out the cards to five students, who must stand in front of the class and arrange themselves in the proper order to produce the sentence, *Where is the bathroom?* Then, I'll call up one more student, and hand her a card that says, *Can you tell me*. Students then have to rearrange themselves to produce, *Can you tell me where the bathroom is?* This helps them see how word order changes when questions are embedded.

Erica Ashton, ESL Teacher

many years of experience). Additionally, a fragment can be a dependent clause that is not embedded within an independent clause (*since the research was funded by the government*). To fix a fragment, students can (a) supply a subject, (b) supply a predicate, or (c) embed the dependent clause in an independent clause, like in the examples below in (26):

(26) a. Dr. Park <u>found no relationship between the two variables</u>.
　　　b. <u>The researchers from the institute with many years of experience</u> visited our lab.
　　　c. <u>Since the research was funded by the government</u> they were able to complete the project.

5.7 Movement

Thus far we have covered simple sentences (independent clauses) and sentences with embedded, dependent clauses. However, some sentences are complex not because they are particularly long, but because there is internal **movement** associated with them. For example, questions are derived from statements. What does this mean? It means that in order to form a question, the original statement must be reshuffled. In other words, the structure of questions are actually declarative statements in a different order. Consider the questions in (27).

(27) a. Are you going to the dinner party?
　　　b. Should we drive there together?
　　　c. What are you bringing?
　　　d. When did you have time to make that?

The first two examples are yes-no questions, or questions that can be answered with a yes or a no. The second two are wh-questions, or questions that require more of an answer. In all four cases, the questions in (27) are actually derived from their declarative counterpart, as in (28).

(28) a. You are going to the dinner party.
　　　b. We should drive there together.
　　　c. You are bringing ___. (*a soufflé*)
　　　d. You had time to make that ___. (*this morning*)

As you can see, the statements in (28) are basically the questions in (27) where the word order has been changed. In some languages, all you need to do in order to form a question is to change the intonation or fill in the blank with a question word like *what* or *when* and the question would be complete.

In languages like English and many European languages, however, question formation requires movement. For instance, in English to derive a question from the statement *you are going to the dinner party*, the auxiliary *are* must be moved to the front of the sentence: *are you going to the dinner party?*

Similarly, the statement *we should drive there together* can be turned into a question by identifying the auxiliary and moving it to the front of the sentence; in this case, *should* is the auxiliary, resulting in the question *should we drive there together?*

For wh-questions, there is an extra step. We still identify the auxiliary and move it to the front of the sentence, like this:

(29)   Are you ~~are~~ bringing ___

Next, we fill in the blank with a wh-word. Since food items are inanimate, we fill it with the wh-word *what*.

(30)   Are you ~~are~~ bringing <u>what</u>

Finally, we have to move the wh-word to the front of the sentence to complete the wh-question.

(31)   What are you ~~are~~ bringing ~~what~~

It is no wonder that this is an area of difficulty for many learners. Constructing a question is much more than simply putting *what* at the beginning of the sentence. The movement involved adds to the complexity of the structure.

Another type of sentence that requires movement in its derivation is a sentence with a passive voice wherein the agent, or the doer of the action, is placed at the end of the clause so that the action and the result of that action are highlighted. Compare the two sentences in (32).

(32)   a. Harry broke the expensive vase.
       b. The expensive vase was broken by Harry.

In the first example, there is an emphasis on the agent; you could almost picture someone pointing a finger at Harry while uttering that sentence. This sentence is in active voice. However, in the second sentence, the agent is displaced, and the focus is on the action and the result. The agent *Harry* is added on at the end in a *by*-phrase. The convenient fact of the *by*-phrase is that it is now optional, so it can be omitted and it would be a perfectly grammatical sentence: *The expensive vase was broken.*

To derive a passive sentence from an active sentence, we follow three stages. First, identify the direct object, or the entity that was acted upon, and move it to the front of the sentence. In this case, that direct object is the noun phrase [*the expensive vase*].

(33)   [The expensive vase] Harry broke ~~the expensive vase~~.

Next, convert the verb to the *be* + past participle form. In this case, *broke* becomes *was broken.*

(34) [The expensive vase] Harry *was broken* ~~the expensive vase~~.

Finally, identify the subject, put it in a *by*-phrase, and move it to the end of the sentence.

(35) [The expensive vase] ~~Harry~~ *was broken* ~~the expensive vase~~ [by Harry].

The end result is the passive voice version *The expensive vase was broken by Harry*. Or, of course, we can leave out the agent altogether and leave the action blameless. Passive voice is used in academic writing to deemphasize the doer of the action and avoid first person. It can also be a handy trick when you want to shift blame or avoid blatantly mentioning the agent in a delicate situation, such as in a court of law.

It is sometimes difficult for learners to recognize passive voice construction because the agent may or may not be present. Additionally, the difference between the verb in an active voice construction and a verb in a passive voice construction is very slight in some languages. Forming the passive is even more challenging because of all the movement involved, where the object becomes the subject and the subject gets moved to a prepositional phrase at the end of the sentence. Derivations such as these might be intuitive to the proficient or native speaker, but to learners there are a lot of moving parts that can lead to difficulty. In the next section, we discuss what teachers can do to address these difficulties.

5.8 Application to Teaching and Learning

Let us take a step back and reconsider why syntax is important. Earlier in this chapter, we talked about how sentences are not a random jumble of words. If we learned ten Gujarati words—a mix of nouns, verbs, prepositions, and a few connectors—would we be able to form a sentence in Gujarati? With the exception of our Gujarati readers, the rest of us would not. That is because we would not know how to string those words together; to be more precise, we do not know the phrase structure rules for Gujarati, so we would not know what the word order is. Because phrase structure rules differ from language to language, word orders differ from language to language as well.

This is the reason why word-for-word translation does not work. For instance, to say *we tried to take the bus but we missed it* in Spanish is *intentamos tomar el autobús pero lo perdimos*. However, if we translate that sentence back to English word-for-word, it sounds nonsensical: *intended to take the bus but it we missed*. If we translate the equivalent sentence from Korean word-for-word, it sounds even stranger: *bus ride did try missed*. Often, beginner language learners will apply the word order of their first or dominant language to the target language, resulting in what sounds ungrammatical. This is quite understandable; students have to wrap their minds around the fact that the language they are learning sometimes works in an entirely different way, and it takes time to get accustomed to the new rules. For example, if you have spoken a subject-verb-object (SVO) language all your life, learning a language that has subject-object-verb (SOV) word order can be challenging. Rather than saying *I ate an apple*, the student has to become familiar and comfortable with the order *I an apple ate* in the target language. It is helpful for teachers to recognize the differences in phrase structure and word order between the students' language and the target language in order to help students overcome some of these barriers.

Another example is that in many of the world's languages, the subject pronoun is not always necessary: it can be omitted if it is understood from context. In other words, if we have been talking about a person named Joe, you don't have to repeat *he* again and again: *Went to the store. When got there, bought some ice cream. Ate it.* While this sounds awkward in English, this is perfectly grammatical and actually preferred in other languages. Languages that allow for the subject pronoun to be omitted are called **prodrop languages**, or sometimes **subject drop** or **null-subject languages**. Prodrop languages have phrase structure rules that make the subject optional. However, students who speak a non-prodrop language tend to have difficulty with intentionally leaving out a subject pronoun because they are accustomed to supplying a subject in every clause. Again, students have the difficult task of learning a new set of phrase structure rules, and the errors they make might be a result of applying the rules of their first or dominant language to the target language.

The two preceding examples are just a tiny sampling of the kinds of challenges students may face when learning another language. As language teachers, how do we help students with these grammatical differences? One strategy is to focus learners' attention to the specific grammatical form you want to target by giving students tasks that require the use of these structures. For example, suppose students are having difficulty with English question formation. While students might easily understand that the wh-word needs to appear in the front of the sentence, they might not remember that the auxiliary verb also needs to move to the front of the sentence right after the wh-word. This is indeed an area that is difficult not just for ESL students but children learning English as their first language because of all the complexity involved. While it can be helpful to explicitly point out that this is how questions are formed in English, often this is not necessarily very effective. For younger learners, it might also not be plausible that they understand such a technical point in the grammar. Instead, teachers can provide tasks where using wh-questions would naturally occur.

One strategy teachers can use is pairing up students to interview one another and write up a biography about their partner. They would have to use wh-questions during the interview such as *Where were you born? What is your birthday? What are your hobbies? Who is your best friend? When did you come to the U.S.?*

There are several things to note with this strategy. The first is that students are not just given these questions by the teacher; they must generate their own questions (with teacher guidance) that utilize the structure they are learning. Anyone can mimic, but it requires cognitive effort to apply the rule for meaningful use. Secondly, it's important to vary the structure so that they are not using the same formula with the same words. *Where were you born, what is your birthday*, etc. are all wh-questions with a fronted wh-word and auxiliaries that are raised, but the wh-word is varied and the auxiliaries are different (*were, are, is, did*). Students get the opportunity to try out different combinations, ensuring that the rule is generative, not static. Lastly, by incorporating the structure you want students to learn in an activity that could generate real interest (asking questions to a peer and getting real responses is fun; asking questions for a computer microphone to record you is not), the student is participating in a meaningful exercise that can be engaging.

Another strategy that can be helpful for learners is to use syntactic knowledge to break down complex academic texts. While general texts tend to be fairly straight forward, academic texts are a genre of their own. They are typically dense and wordy, often containing complex modifiers and embedded clauses. The average spoken sentence is about seven words long, but an average written academic sentence is about twenty words long. One way to help learners deal with a complex sentence is to partition it into smaller pieces. Take the sentence in (36) as an example.

(36) Mosses and other bryophytes are distinguished from algae by several features derived during evolutionary adaptation to living on land.

(Campbell & Reece, 2002, p. 576)

While the sentence is informative and well-constructed, language learners would most likely have difficulty with this sentence. Certainly, the vocabulary can be a hindrance; native speakers also have difficulty with new academic vocabulary such as *bryophytes*. However, what may be an additional challenge to a learner of English is that this sentence has passive construction and embedded clauses. Recognizing this is helpful because you can help students focus on the most important content in the sentence. First, we learned earlier that in passive sentences, there is often a *by*-phrase that is optional. Let us identify that *by*-phrase and omit it.

(37) Mosses and other bryophytes are distinguished from algae ~~by several features derived during evolutionary adaptation to living on land~~.

Omitting the optional *by*-phrase in a passive sentence allows us to focus on the main clause, which is much easier to digest. The clause *mosses and other bryophytes are distinguished from algae* is simpler to tackle without the *by*-phrase here. Next, the *by*-phrase can be further broken down by identifying the relative clause, which is bracketed in (38).

(38) by several features [derived during evolutionary adaptation to living on land]

The relative clause is a modifier for the noun *features*. Thus, everything in the bracket helps explain a little more about the features. If we want to dissect it a little more, you could pinpoint some of the prepositional phrases that are tucked inside the relative clause.

(39) derived [during evolutionary adaptation [to living [on land]]]

Each of these prepositional phrases are embedded within another. It may sound more academic than something like *on big plates with loads of food*, but in truth the structure is exactly the same. Both would have the exact same tree diagrams. After that, the sentence is not so intimidating.

Recommended Website

A free online tree diagram website
   http://mshang.ca/syntree/

Notes

1. *Ran out the door* is a verb followed by a prepositional phrase, while *found out* is a phrasal verb followed by the noun phrase *the truth*.
2. Determiners do have phrases, but for the purposes of this chapter, we will leave them be. There are definitely such things as determiner phrases (DP) that you might explore if you study syntax further.

Further Reading

Carnie, A. (2012). *Syntax: A generative introduction*. Hoboken, NJ: John Wiley & Sons.
Huddleston, R., & Pullum, G. K. (2005). *A student's introduction to English grammar*. Cambridge, UK: Cambridge University Press.
Larsen-Freeman, D., & Celce-Murcia, M. (2015). *The grammar book: Form, meaning, and use for English language teachers*. Boston, MA: Heinle ELT.

Exercises

1. For each of the sentences below, identify the **part of speech** of the underlined word(s). Then, give one piece of evidence to support your choice.

   a. Jillian and her sister Suzanne are planning a trip to Chicago.
   b. They often like to travel together.
   c. Suzanne wants to visit the museums.
   d. Jillian would like to go on an architecture tour.
   e. They found a good price for tickets to a show as well.

2. Identify the type of phrase. Then, draw a tree diagram for each phrase. Hint: some phrases may have embedded phrases within them.

    a. my class
    b. in the snow
    c. caught the ball
    d. this interesting research
    e. very slow
    f. very slowly
    g. finding a new assistant for our department
    h. kindly helped the students with their homework

3. Diagram the following sentences.

    a. Garrett found his keys.
    b. The book was interesting.
    c. Those nice folks recommended this restaurant.

4. The following sentence has two different interpretations. What are those interpretations? Draw a tree diagram for each interpretation.

    a. I tickled the bear with a feather.

5. Embedded questions are a type of dependent clause that is embedded within an independent clause. They are similar to regular wh-questions, but are slightly different in terms of movement. How is the embedded question different from the main clause question?

    a. Main question: Who are you calling?
        Embedded question: I don't know who you are calling.

    b. Main question: What should we order?
        Embedded question: They told me what we should order.

    c. Main question: How does she know?
        Embedded question: I wonder how she knows?

Reference

Campbell, N. A., & Reece, J. B. (2002). *Biology* (6th ed.). New York: Pearson.

6 Semantics and Pragmatics
The Study of Meanings

6.1 Introduction

In the last several chapters, we have been building up language from the smallest component all the way to complex sentences. We have learned how to structure sounds and words, phrases, and clauses. However, what is structure without meaning? To explore this question, let us consider a famous sentence in (1).

(1) Colorless green ideas sleep furiously.

While the sentence is structurally sound and grammatically correct, there are some problems with the meaning. We might point out that something colorless cannot also be green, that ideas cannot be colored, that ideas do not sleep, and that sleeping cannot be done furiously. This sentence demonstrates that even if you follow all the phrase structure rules of a language—in fact, you can probably diagram this sentence after reading Chapter 5—it can still yield a meaningless utterance. Thus, it is not enough that a language learner acquire the structures in the target language; the learner must also understand (1) meanings of individual words, (2) how words function together in phrases and clauses to make meaning, and (3) how the speaker and listener make sense of this through context, norms, and other non-linguistics elements. Semantics is the layer of language that provides this understanding.

In this chapter, we will begin by discussing **lexical semantics,** or how meaning is created within and between words. Next, we will describe how meaning is derived from phrases and sentences. This chapter also discusses how non-grammatical factors such as speaker attitudes and situational context contribute to meaning. It explains how meaning is communicated in conversation and shows that what people say and how they say things are culturally conditioned (cross-cultural pragmatics). Finally, we will provide some strategies for helping learners to use language in culturally appropriate ways.

6.2 Lexical Semantics

6.2.1 Sense and Reference

Let us begin with a single word. Meaning can be constructed in many ways, but at the word level, it comes down to two things: **sense** and **reference**. Sense is defined as the concept or mental representation of a word. If you hear the word *bird*, you might imagine a feathered and winged animal. Reference, however, is the relation between the linguistic expression and the existence of that entity in the real world. You might look outside and see a bird, and that feathered and winged animal you see is matched up with the verbal expression [br̩d]. Since birds are both conceptual and real—and most people have seen one—the word [br̩d] has both sense and reference.

It is possible for words to have different senses but the same reference. Look at the underlined words in the following sentences.

(2) a. <u>My brother</u> likes tacos.
     b. <u>Jason</u> likes tacos.
     c. <u>He</u> likes tacos.

The words *my brother, Jason,* and *he* are all different in sense, conjuring up different mental representations: *my brother* is a familial relation, *Jason* is a name, and *he* is a masculine singular pronoun. However, they all refer to the same person in this case. It's also possible to have the same sense but different references, as in the sentence below in (3).

(3) <u>This little piggy</u> went to market; <u>this little piggy</u> went home.

In this segment from a children's nursery rhyme, the subject of both clauses is *this little piggy*, which both have the same sense; both conjure up the image of a small pig. However, in this context there are two references, or two piggies, and they went in two different directions. In fact, the nursery rhyme is recited with emphasis on the word *this* to indicate that there are indeed two different piggies. Thus, it is possible to have one sense and multiple references.

Are there words in language that have only one or the other? In other words, can you have a concept of something (sense) but not have an example of that meaning in the real world (reference)? Certainly. A dragon, for example, has sense: you can picture a large, scaly creature with wings that breathes fire. However, it does not have an actual referent in the real world as it is a fictional animal; thus, it does not have reference. In reverse, you could experience something in the real world (reference) but not have a word or expression for it (sense), at least in the languages you know. In this case, it has reference but not sense.

Language learners, especially younger students, tend to find words with reference much easier to learn than words without reference. Babies learning their first language often start with words of family members or common items around the house, in large part because the referent is immediately present and readily available. For second language learners, this is also the case. When first learning a new language, most teachers start with vocabulary pertaining to tangible objects around the room, or common greetings that can immediately be put to use. Older students learning a word without a reference might access a translation to learn the new word in the target language; even if a dragon does not exist in the world, there is a word for it in their other language and you already have the concept of a dragon in your head. But if you have never even seen a picture of a dragon, learning the meaning of that word without the reference or sense tends to be more of a challenge.

6.2.2 Word Relations

We learned in Chapter 5 that words are grouped into structural units called constituents. Linguists have also learned that words are grouped into meaning units as well. When learning a list of vocabulary, learners tend to do better when they learn the words grouped into categories. Some semantic categories we will discuss here are **synonyms**, **antonyms**, and **hyper-/hyponyms**.

Synonyms are words that are similar in meaning. Some examples of synonym pairs are *trash-garbage, eat-consume, beautiful-lovely, watch-look*. We are careful not to say synonyms have identical meanings. In fact, words in languages tend not to be redundant. Even if there is a word that seems almost interchangeable with the other, there tends to be small nuanced differences. Let us take trash and garbage, for example. In American English, trash and garbage tend to be used by similar groups of people; in other words, it is not necessarily a dialectal difference, where some regions prefer the word *trash* and other regions use *garbage*. A single speaker might use both words. That single speaker might swear there is really no difference for them. However, does it truly have the same exact meaning for that person? A *trash can* and a *garbage can* might yield different senses and references (Is one metal? Is one kept inside the home whereas the other is outside?). *Trash disposal* versus *garbage disposal* might conjure up different images as well. The adjective forms *trashy* versus *garbagy* might also be different. Many people realize there are minute differences that can be teased apart when you take some time to analyze your own language use. Synonyms are thus words that have similar meanings, but it is challenging to find two words within the same language that have the exact same meaning and use.

Antonyms are words that have opposite meanings. There are four types of antonyms: complementary antonyms, gradable antonyms, reverse antonyms, and relational antonyms. Complementary antonyms are words that are direct opposites of the other, where typically one falls under one category or the other: X vs. not X. Such a pair would be *alive-dead*, where *dead* means not *alive*. Other complementary antonyms include pairs such as *married-unmarried, mortal-immortal*, and *on-off*. Gradable antonyms are words whose meanings fall on opposite sides of a spectrum, but there are in between states between the two words. An example of a pair of gradable antonym is *big* and *small*, in which the two words indicate opposite meanings on a spectrum of different sizes. Other examples of gradable antonyms include *hot-cold, light-dark*, and *happy-sad*. Reverse antonyms are words whose meanings suggest movement, and one word undoes the other movement, like *right-left, push-pull*, or *break-fix*. Finally, relational antonyms are opposite words whose meaning only exists if the other exists. Such an example is *teacher* and *student*, where teacher cannot exist without any students to teach, and one cannot be a student without a teacher of some sort. Other examples of relational antonyms are *borrow-lend* and *over-under*.

There are many words where a true polar opposite does not exist or is debatable. What is the antonym of *dog*? A student might say *cat*, because culturally, we think of them as pets that do not get along (not always true) but both are common household domesticated mammals and have many similarities—perhaps more similarities than there are differences. Even more tricky is identifying an antonym for a verb. For instance, what is the antonym of *run*? Is it to stand? Sit? Walk? This might differ depending on the context. For instance, in the context of running a marathon, the opposite would be to *not* run a marathon, in which case you could be standing still or sitting. Antonyms for adjectives, adverbs, and prepositions tend to be easier because they tend to take on a modifying role, but it tends to become more open to debate when it comes to identifying antonyms for verbs.

The last two word relations are actually antonyms themselves: hypernyms and hyponyms. Hypernyms are superordinate words that form a set or category in which other specific words fall under. For instance, *color* is a hypernym of the word *green*, because *color* is the set or category for specific words such as *green*. Hyponyms are words with a specific meaning that falls under a general category or set. The word *green* is a hyponym of *color*, because *green* is a specific word that belongs under the category of *color*. Some other examples of hypernym-hyponym pairs are *clothing-socks, insect-ant*, and *move-run*.

6.2.3 Homophony and Polysemy

In many of the world's languages, there are areas of ambiguity that stem from a lack of one-to-one correspondence between words and the meanings represented by them. We discussed in Chapter 2 that in English, some letters make more than one sound, and some sounds are represented by more than one letter. Meaning works the same way. **Homophony**, or the phenomenon in which multiple words with different meanings have the same pronunciation, causes difficulty for learners, native and nonnative alike. For example, in English the words *two, too*, and *to* are challenging because they are pronounced the same way but mean three different things. In spoken language, one can easily disambiguate these based on context, but in writing learners have the task of corresponding the right meaning with the right spelling.

Even more challenging still is **polysemy**, in which one word can have multiple meanings. An example of polysemy in English is *duck*, where one meaning is a noun for a water bird and another is a verb referring to the act of quickly lowering one's head. Other examples of polysemy include *fire* (set *fire* to something; *fire* an employee), *cast* (wear a *cast* on my arm; the *cast* of *Cheers*; *cast* a spell; *cast* something aside), or *stick* (a tree *stick; stick* a note on the door; *stick* the landing). While proficient speakers can usually figure out the intended meaning based on context, learners of the language have trouble with polysemy. This is because learners tend to learn first the most common definition of a word. For instance, when a learner hears the word *stick*, probably the most likely meaning they have in mind is a stick from a tree. They may not have heard *stick* being used as a verb to mean attach, and most assuredly they are probably not familiar with the very specific usage as in *stick the landing*.

However, a surprising number of academic jargon is polysemic, and it typically has very specific meanings. Some examples are *class, report, board,* or *subject. Class,* for example, is a high-frequency word that beginners might know to mean a group of students learning together. They might even learn that it can be modified with the subject, like *math class, music class,* etc. and that it can be used as a vocative to address the students (e.g., *good morning, class*). However, *class* can also mean a body of students whose year of graduation is the same (*the class of '02*) or level in school (*sophomore class*), which have slightly different nuanced uses. Even more technical still, *class* can refer to one's socioeconomic level, and it can also signify etiquette or polished behavior (e.g., *to have class*). *Class* can also be a specific word in biological taxonomy just below *phylum,* or it can be a word signifying a set of variables in mathematics. These are just the nouns. Disambiguating such a word and knowing which meaning is being employed is a challenging task. Academic texts are full of such specific uses, where polysemy can often cause difficulties for language learners.

This is one of the pitfalls of dictionaries. While looking up a word is a simple mechanical task, trying to figure out which definition is being used requires a basic understanding of each definition. More difficult still is then producing that word in the right context. To go one step further, dictionaries may not always provide the true meaning of something. Recall in Chapter 1, we explored the meaning of *red* versus *red-red,* and how that second term implies a prototype for a meaning. *Red-red* is not something you can look up in a dictionary. This brings us to the question, what does it mean to know a word? While most might say it means knowing the definition of that word, we have learned that it goes beyond just the definition. What teachers often focus on is students understanding and having a large breadth of vocabulary knowledge; the more words you know, the better. However, we might argue that to truly crack the lexical semantics layer, you also need to have depth of vocabulary: knowing all the layers of meaning one word can have (e.g., *class*) and also understanding the usage.

6.3 Phrasal Semantics

Meaning does not stop at the word boundary, of course. Meaning can be constructed and construed at the phrasal or sentence level, a subfield referred to as **phrasal semantics**. A word's relationship to the other words around it, as well as the role within the constituent, is an important part of phrasal semantics. This is where semantics interfaces with syntax. **Semantic roles** (or sometimes called **thematic or theta roles**) are the functions that a predicate can assign to the various constituents around them. For instance, let us take a verb like *hit*. Such a predicate requires two entities: the entity that does the hitting (X), and the entity that is hit (Y).

(4)   X hit Y.

Entities that are capable of doing the hitting are usually animate. We call these doers of actions, or *agents*. The entity that gets hit—animate or inanimate—is the target of the action. These undergoers of action are called *patients*. Agent and patient are semantic roles. In a sentence like *Jane hit the baseball*, the agent is *Jane* and the patient is *the baseball*.

Different predicates require different semantic roles. Some examples of these semantic roles can be seen in Table 6.1. In a predicate like *to fall*, for instance, there is not an active causer of the action; usually, falling is incidental. Thus, the entity that did the falling is neither an agent nor a patient, but an *experiencer*. X experienced falling.

(5)   X fell.

In a sentence like *The child fell*, the experiencer is *the child*. The predicate *fall* also does not require a direct object, so you cannot have a sentence like *The child fell the chair*.

Table 6.1 Semantic Roles

Semantic Role	Definition	Example
Agent	Doer of the action or event	*Andrew* kicked the ball.
Patient	Undergoer of the action or event	Andrew kicked *the ball*.
Experiencer	Living entity that experiences the action or event	*Andrew* fell on the ice.
Instrument	Entity used to accomplish the action or event	Andrew hit the ball with *a bat*.
Theme	Entity that is moved by the action or event	Andrew sent *a message*.
Source	Location or entity that something moves from	Andrew left *the house*.
Goal	Location or entity that something moves to	Andrew went to *school*.
Benefactive	Entity that benefits from the action or event	Andrew gave *me* a gift.

Why are these semantic roles important? Learning about semantic roles shows how predicates are all quite different in their requirements. All of these words are verbs—think, kick, send, read—but they have different requirements for what can be its subject and what can be its object, if any. Remember our nonsensical sentence *colorless green ideas sleep furiously*? For the verb *sleep*, you cannot have that subject be a inanimate noun (e.g., ideas); *sleep* requires an experiencer as its subject, and ideas cannot experience. Even if you have a perfectly grammatical sentence that is syntactically sound and follows all the phrase structure rules, if you disobey the semantic roles the predicate requires, the sentence won't make any sense:

(6)   The carpet thinks.
(7)   A window kicked the man.
(8)   Fear sent the tree my mother.
(9)   Clarification read a book.

Certainly, musicians, poets, and other literary minds can intentionally flout those semantic roles for rhetoric intent. A beautiful sentence like *the sea whispered secrets to the wind* breaks the semantic roles required of the verb *whisper*. However, to be able to intentionally bend these rules, the user must first understand what those rules are. And outside of these highly specialized uses, semantic role requirements must be followed.

Closely related to semantic roles is what is known as **transitivity**, a property that predicates can have that determine whether or not it has a direct object. Predicates can be transitive, intransitive, or ditransitive. **Transitive** predicates, such as *hit*, require a direct object. When transitive predicates appear with no direct object, they sound awkward: *I hit*. In contrast, **intransitive** predicates, such as *fall*, require no direct object. Intransitive predicates sound awkward when a direct object does appear, such as *The child fell the chair*. Ditransitive predicates are ones in which two objects are required: a direct object and an indirect object. An example of a ditransitive predicate is the verb *give*, as in *I gave my mother a gift*, where the NP [*my mother*] is the indirect object with the semantic role of "benefactive", and the NP [*a gift*] is the direct object with the semantic role of "theme".

The neat thing about semantics and semantic roles is that you can make sense of it in the real world. It follows that you cannot hit unless you have something to hit (otherwise, it's not a hit; it's a miss). Falling is something that just happens to someone or something, however. You can cause something to fall, but you would use a different verb or construction (I pushed, knocked down, etc. or I made it fall). And when you *give*, you have the item you are giving and the person or entity you are giving it to. If you are standing there holding a gift but it hasn't reached the recipient, you haven't *given* it yet.

6.4 Pragmatics

So far we have discussed how meaning is created at the morpheme level (*happy* → *happily*), word level (*duck* vs. *duck*), and phrase level (*Vincent sent a letter*). In this section, we talk about how meaning is created through use and context, a branch of linguistics called pragmatics. Meaning can be generated and inferred not just through our knowledge of the sense and reference of a word or how that word is used in a phrase, but also our knowledge about the situational context and our knowledge about culture.

6.4.1 Context

The context of when, how, and with whom language is used is an important layer of language. Think about a phrase that would be perfectly appropriate in one setting, and awkward or rude in another. Think about the way you would speak in a job interview versus how you might speak to your closest friend. It is not enough to simply utter well-formed utterances; you have to understand the situation and setting and know what is appropriate for that circumstance.

Context can change the meaning of a single word. The word *okay* might be defined in a dictionary as a statement of consent, agreement, or a description. But how you say it, when you say it, and who you say it to can drastically change that meaning. Try saying the word *okay* to convey the following meanings with different contexts:

(10) You are uncertain about what just happened
(11) You want to seem dispassionate but you are actually very excited about an offer
(12) Someone makes a rude comment
(13) A child tells you something inane and you have to pretend to be impressed

A single word can have dozens of meanings, and the tone of how you say it paired with the context can change it from one meaning to another.

Meaning can also be created and inferred through different situational contexts. Every sentence in the following conversations are well-formed and are perfectly fine in isolation. However, given the context, they are inappropriate or awkward. See (14).

(14)

    a. Laura: Hey, John, can I talk to you about something?
       John: I'll see you later.

    b. Teacher: John, can you close that window, please?
       John: Yes, I can. [does nothing]

    c. CEO: Good morning, Mr. Sullivan, thank you for coming in for an interview.
       John: No prob, kiddo.

The first conversation in (14a) is awkward because Laura seems to want to talk to John about something serious, and John responds with a farewell greeting.

The immediate rejection is potentially hurtful to Laura and awkward to the overhearer. In the second conversation in (14b), the teacher is asking John to close the window, framing it in a question with the modal *can* to be polite (as opposed to simply ordering him to close the window: *John, close the window*). However, the response is quite awkward because John responds by saying he can close the window, possibly interpreting it as a question of whether he has the physical capacity to close it, and does not actually perform the action. In (14c), the CEO of the company with whom John is interviewing addresses John in a formal way, using the salutation *Mr. Sullivan*. However, John responds in an informal manner, calling the CEO *kiddo* and using the phrase *no prob*, both of which would be perfectly fine in some contexts but unusual in a job interview. In all three cases, John's (non)response is rude or awkward because he does not understand or misreads the situational context. It is also possible he does understand the situational context and is responding in this manner to be intentionally discourteous.

The point here is that meaning is not just words and phrases; it's understanding the how, who, and why of your surrounding context. This is something that young children sometimes take a while to learn. A child might have excellent syntax and phonology, but it is not for several years later that the child develops awareness of what is pragmatically appropriate or inappropriate. You might have heard a child ask an awkward question or say something loudly in a public place that might be construed as inappropriate or awkward had it been an adult speaker. Often times, when a young child does something like this, people are pretty forgiving. However, the same courtesy is not granted when it is a language learner, especially if the learner is older. Pragmatic competence is language-specific, so what is considered appropriate does not necessarily translate from one language to another. Thus, pragmatic competence is something language learners need to focus on and learn explicitly. Teachers can help learners practice this by giving them fictional contexts, such as in the *okay* exercise above, and responding with the same word with various intonations. Teachers can also provide students with example conversations where something has gone awry and ask students to identify what went wrong and how to fix it.

6.4.2 Culture

Related to the foregoing discussion, culture and cultural context can factor into meaning. One might assume that what is pragmatically acceptable in one culture is the same in another, but if you ever travel to another country or region, you will quickly notice that this is not the case. What is taboo in one area—whether that be religion, age, job, death—is not necessarily the case in another area.

Take apologizing, for example. In your most familiar culture, what would be the appropriate apology, if any, if you are standing in a crowded bus or

Voices From the Classroom 6.1 — Formality and Audience

With an increased use of technology in classrooms and overall student life, teacher and student communication has shifted from in-person interactions to more emails and internet platform messaging. This being said, I work with students on email formatting including appropriate greetings, wording, and formatting depending on audience. I introduce levels of formality, which may differ in their native countries, and provide examples of emails directed to employers, supervisors, teachers, and peers. I've found that it is a low risk opportunity for code switching and kids are able to double check that what they're trying to say is actually what they're writing down.

Gabriela Melendez, High School Bilingual Teacher

train and you accidentally and lightly bump up against someone you do not know? In one culture, it might be normal to say quietly *sorry* without making eye contact and without need for response. In another culture, you might have to say *oops, sorry about that!* and the other person has to say something like *no problem!*, which might lead to some comment about how the bus is especially crowded today. In other cultures, no apology is necessary, and verbally apologizing would actually be an annoyance or embarrassment to the other person.

The same range of pragmatic appropriateness applies for complimenting. In some cultures, it is polite and expected to compliment someone. Among people in the U.S., for example, it is not uncommon for one person to compliment the other on a clothing item or accessory (*I love your earrings*) as a generic conversation starter or signal of openness and friendliness, even if the speaker is not necessarily interested in the particular item. In other parts of the world, it would be highly embarrassing to point out what someone is wearing. More interesting yet is the expected response: in some cultures you would downplay the value of the thing you were complimented on (*oh, this old thing? It's old and falling apart*), in others you would explain in great detail where you got it, especially if it was acquired through a particularly good deal, and in other cultures you would be expected to gift the item to the complimenter. Again, the take home point is that meanings for what might seem grammatically the same thing (*I like your watch*) are determined culturally and can change drastically from *I'm being friendly* to *Give me your watch*.

> **Voices From the Classroom 6.2—Teaching Pragmatics in the Language Classroom**
>
> Sean Stinson, who teaches ESOL in an elementary school, uses pragmatics for both language acquisition and classroom management. He emphasizes the vocabulary of politeness and teaches formulaic expressions such as *excuse me, please,* and *thank you* early on to newcomers and low fluency learners. He then moves on to other expressions necessary to move conversations along such as *That's interesting, I'd like to add . . .* or *That's an interesting answer, but I think . . .* while at the same time urging students not to interrupt each other. Sean teaches more advanced students that the past tense is considered more polite, as in *I was wondering . . . .* In a communicative context, learners are acquiring cultural and language competencies. At the same time, Sean is creating a learning environment where trial and error, thinking out loud, and peer support are encouraged.
>
> Owen Andrews, Adult ESL Teacher

6.4.3 Attitude and Perspective

Meaning can also be determined through the attitude of the speaker or listener. One's attitude, preconceived notion, perspective, and other nonlinguistic psychological states can change the meaning of a particular utterance or the interpretation of an utterance. For example, you can hear an identical word said exactly the same way in different ways depending on your point of view. You may have experienced a time where you and another person heard the same thing but had two very different interpretations. Perhaps you thought the speaker was kind and welcoming, while your friend thought the speaker was rude and pretentious. The attitude and perspective of the speaker and listener can inject meaning that transcends grammatical structure. Likewise, preconceived notions can alter one's perception of meaning. If two people with very different ideals listen to the same political speech, for instance, the person whose values align with the politician might evaluate the speaker as astute, clear, and provocative while the person whose values differ from the politician may believe that the speaker was obtuse, unintelligible, and unoriginal.

An empirical example of this comes from a study by Rubin (1992). The researcher investigated undergraduate students' perceptions of their instructors based on physical appearance. In one part of the study, Rubin played an audio of a recorded lecture by a woman—a native speaker of English—to one group of students while projecting a still picture of a Caucasian woman on the screen in the front of the room. Then, the students were asked various questions about the clarity, effectiveness, and speaking ability of the audio lecture. Students thought that the woman was clear, easy-to-understand, and seemed generally positive about the lecture. Then, Rubin played the identical audio file to another group of students, but this time he displayed a photo of an Asian woman on the screen. Students were asked the same questions, but this time students overall thought the lecture was not as effective, and some of the students said that the lecture was hard to understand because of the woman's accent. Keep in mind, of course, that it was the same audio recorded by a native English speaker that the first group of students heard. It appeared from the study that students actually heard an accent where there wasn't one. Generally, students in the group with the Asian woman's photo felt that the lecture was not as good. This suggests that even when two people—or two groups of people—hear the exact same thing, the meaning and overall impression can change given their perception of the speaker. By simply changing out the image of the person who they assumed was the speaker (even though that information was not given), the listeners received different meanings and had different experiences of listening to the lecture.

It's important to understand this as a language teacher and educator in general. Try as they might, teachers do not always have the same attitudes toward every student. Often times, students that are quieter might seem like they do not have as much language competence, while others that are more outwardly vocal seem like they are taking more risks and developing the language more effectively. Sometimes, teachers might have less patience with students that act out in class, and that might alter how they judge that student's true language ability. It takes a careful eye and conscious effort to discern that your attitude toward an idea, a situation, or another person might be affecting the meaning you take away from that person.

6.4.4 Having Effective Conversation: Grice's Maxims

We have discussed how meaning can be altered based on elements outside of phonology, morphology, or syntax, such as through context, culture, and attitude. Paul Grice, a British philosopher of language, is best known for his "**cooperative principle**", which describes how people achieve effective conversational communication in social situations. According to Grice, listeners and speakers act cooperatively and accept one another to be understood in a particular way. Grice's Maxims of Conversation take these into account, but also suggest a set of guidelines that, when followed, tend to have good results in human conversation. The four rules are as follows:

Maxim of quality: be truthful
Maxim of quantity: be as informative as required, no more than is adequate
Maxim of relevance: be as relevant as possible
Maxim of manner: be orderly and clear, do not be ambiguous

The **maxim of quality** suggests that generally, you should tell the truth or what you know to be true. When you take a French class, you should be able to assume that what your French teacher is teaching you is actually French. Or, if someone asks you on the street which way it is to the bus stop, you ought to point them to the actual direction of the bus stop rather than intentionally pointing them in the opposite direction. Grice recommends that generally people tell the truth or what they believe to be the truth.

The **maxim of quantity** advises that you be as informative as is required, but provide no more than what is adequate. In other words, we strive to say enough but not too much. For instance, if you are at a restaurant with a friend and he asks what you're thinking of ordering for your meal, it is appropriate to respond with a brief description of the two things you are considering, but perhaps not regale the person with why those two choices are specifically superior than all the rest of the food items on the menu. That falls under the category of too much information. On the other hand, if you simply reply to your friend "food", it comes off a bit curt and does not really answer the question adequately. This response is not enough quantity.

The third maxim is the **maxim of relevance**, in which we are recommended to be as on-topic and relevant as possible. In other words, conversations generally go better if one does not hop around topics haphazardly. As an example, if your colleague invites you to a social gathering, a relevant response should have something to do with the invitation, such as *I would love to stop by*, or *I wish I could, I have a prior engagement*, or even *I'm not sure, but thanks for the invite*. It would disobey the maxim of relevance if your response to such an invitation was *It took me forever to get to work this morning!* Or *Did you have lunch yet?*

Lastly, the **maxim of manner** suggests that we be orderly, clear, and avoid ambiguity. In other words, this maxim asks participants in an interaction to not make it extra difficult for the other people involved in the conversation. Consider a scenario in which you are conversing with a small group of people, perhaps to make plans for a weekend. Being orderly might mean you wait for one person to finish an utterance before speaking. Being clear could mean that you articulate your preferences so that everyone understands. Avoiding ambiguity might mean, for example, you use terms of address so people know you're talking to one person versus the whole group: "could I get a ride with you, Melissa?" versus "could I get a ride?"

The maxims of conversation, when unintentionally violated, can result in appearing awkward or clueless at best, offensive or hurtful at worst. However, Grice's maxims are intentionally flouted quite often. This is what results in humor, irony, or sarcasm. Take humor, for example: sitcoms and other comedies are riddled with maxim flouting. The last frame of a comic strip usually incorporates some form of bending the rules of a maxim or two. In a film, every time a blatant untruth is told, a character abruptly changes the topic, or gives an unexpectedly long-winded response, a maxim is being flouted. Maxims are also violated intentionally for purposes of irony or sarcasm, saying the opposite of what you mean or intentionally not giving enough information.

6.4.5 Speech Acts

While we think of actions as being performed through physical action and motion, language can be an action, too. **Speech acts** are actions performed through language. We perform a speech act when we greet, compliment, thank, command, refuse, or ask permission. Speech acts come in five categories: **declaratives, commissives, expressives, representatives**, and **directives**. A declarative speech act changes the world around the speaker. Some examples of a declarative speech act are a *decree* or a *pronouncement*. A commissive speech act affects the speaker and commissions oneself to a course of action: *promise, swear, threat, offer, vow*. An expressive speech act is one in which the speaker expresses one's attitudes or state of affairs. Examples of expressive speech acts include *thank, hate, regret, apologize*. Representative speech acts are assertions or claims that the speaker believes to be true: *assert, believe, conclude, deny*. Finally, directive speech acts are ones where the speaker compels the listener to do something, such as *invite, command, request, warn*.

A special type of speech act across these five categories is what is known as a **performative speech act**. Performative speech acts are ones in which the words themselves are the action. For example, when someone says *I promise*, that promise is happening at the moment of—and through—the words themselves. Without saying the words, the action of promising does not happen. Another example of a performative speech act is when a pronouncement is made. The words *I pronounce* themselves perform the action of pronouncement.

Speech acts are of interest to language teachers and learners because there are multiple ways to accomplish one particular speech act. And like our discussion of culture earlier in this chapter, how you accomplish a speech act can be different from language to language. As an exercise, think of how many different ways you can refuse a dinner invitation. It depends on who the invitation was from, of course, and what the reason was that you could not (or did not want to) attend. The refusal itself could be done with as few words as "sorry, can't make it" to a long drawn out explanation of why you cannot attend and how much you wish you could. Language learners tend to have difficulty with this because there are many cultural and linguistic waters to navigate: different levels of formality, consequences for refusal, expression of regret. In some languages, like English, longer utterances typically sound more polite than shorter utterances, which then disadvantage the language learner.

Another reason why speech acts can be challenging for learners is that the function of the speech act does not always match the syntactic structure. In other words, syntactically speaking, we typically have declarative, interrogative, imperative, and exclamative sentences. Students are generally taught that declarative sentences are statements, interrogative sentences are questions, imperatives are commands, and exclamatives are exclamations.

Table 6.2 Syntax-Speech Act Mismatches

Speech Act	Syntactic Structure	Example Sentence
Question	Declarative	I was wondering if you can come.
Command	Declarative	You will put your shoes on *now*.
Command	Interrogative	Can you please be quiet?
Exclaim	Interrogative	What in the world is this?
Greet	Imperative	Take care.
Offend	Imperative	Don't cook that again anytime soon.
Offend	Exclamative	What a silly outfit!
Greet	Exclamative	What a long time it's been!

However, a declarative speech act does not always utilize declarative syntax, and a questioning speech act does not always appear in the form of a question. In Table 6.2, you will see some examples of these syntax-speech act mismatches.

The trouble with the mismatch is that you do not have a one-to-one correspondence between the speech acts and syntactic structures. However, people tend not to be consciously aware of this, and language learners are rarely taught that there are multiple syntactic structures for one speech act and multiple speech acts for one syntactic structure. The mismatch can be misleading when students are taught that declarative sentences are statements, interrogative sentences are questions, and so on, resulting in possible misinterpretations or missed opportunities for further tools for expression.

To help students understand the differences between speech acts and syntactic structures, choose one speech act, such as *command*, and brainstorm together as many different ways to command someone to do a particular task (e.g., close the door). The brainstorm can include a range of delicately polite to downright offensive ways to command someone, which can also be a lesson on what constitutes rude versus polite rhetoric in the target language. Students can then identify the different syntactic structures used, grouping them together into categories. A discussion of the range of syntactic structures in conjunction with speech acts used may lend itself to discovery about the vast array of syntax that can accomplish the same speech act, but also identify any patterns within the target language (e.g., Does using more words sound more polite? Does commanding someone using a question sound more polite than a straightforward one? Does this differ between the student's dominant language and the target language?).

Further Reading

Löbner, S. (2014). *Understanding semantics*. New York: Routledge.
O'Keeffe, A., Clancy, B., & Adolphs, S. (2019). *Introducing pragmatics in use*. New York: Routledge.

Exercises

1. Identify the following pairs of words as synonyms, antonyms, or hyper/hyponyms. If they are antonyms, name what type they are. If they are hyper/hyponyms, identify which is the hypernym and which is the hyponym.

   a. sink-basin
   b. fork-utensil
   c. clear-opaque
   d. dish-plate
   e. fish-trout
   f. true-false
   g. huge-enormous
   h. in-out
   i. tighten-loosen
   j. tulip-flower
   k. love-hate

2. In each sentence, identify the semantic role of the underlined noun phrase.

   a. <u>Petra</u> scheduled the meeting.
   b. <u>The students</u> studied for the exam.
   c. I sent it to <u>the main office</u>.
   d. Jamie dug a hole with <u>a shovel</u>.
   e. The email was from <u>the dean</u>.
   f. <u>We</u> overheard them talking.
   g. I'm running errands for <u>my sick roommate</u>.
   h. They brought <u>drinks</u> to the picnic.
   i. <u>Jessie</u> saw the snow falling.

3. Technology allows us to have instantaneous conversations through writing. Consider and discuss how punctuation and capitalization changes the meaning of the same word or sentence. How is the punctuation or capitalization in written communication analogous with strategies for conveying meaning in oral communication?

4. Find a 5- to 10-minute clip of a television sitcom. Identify some examples of maxim flouting and discuss how each contribute to the humor of the situation, character, or show.

5. What is the speech act performed by each of the underlined sentences in the following conversation? Classify each speech act into one of the five categories: declaratives, commissives, expressives, representatives, and directives.

   A: <u>Excuse me, do you happen to have the time?</u>
   B: It's 7:45.

A: Okay, thanks. I thought the train was supposed to come at 7:40.
B: Yeah, it's never on time.
A: Oh, really? Ugh, I hope I'm not late to my meeting.
B: Where are you going? Downtown?
A: Yeah, city center. It said it was supposed to take only half an hour, but now I'm worried.
B: Usually it comes no more than like 10 or 15 minutes late. What time's your meeting?
A: At 9 o'clock.
B: Oh, you should be fine.
A: Oh really?
B: Yeah, my office is in city center and I always make it there by like 8:30.
A: Okay, whew.

Reference

Rubin, D. L. (1992). Nonlanguage factors affecting undergraduates' judgments of non-native English-speaking teaching assistants. *Research in Higher Education, 33*(4), 511–531. https://doi.org/10.1007/BF00973770

7 Language in Society

7.1 Introduction

In the previous chapters, we have discussed the nature of language as a human cognitive process governed by rules. However, one of the key reasons why people use language, care about language, get into heated arguments about language, and why so many of us spend time learning language is because of its role in our society. Language is a social tool, a marker of identity, an expression of our ideologies, and a reminder of the communities we live in. Thus, language is intimately tied to our lives and our cultures. In this chapter, we will describe how language is used in social interaction and how speech marks a speaker's social identity. We will explain how speech communities may be distinguished by different sociolinguistic norms, and discuss a variety of factors that contribute to language variation, such as geographical location, social class, gender, and age of the speakers. We will discuss the ways in which language discrimination occurs and how this is linked not to the language itself, but larger underlying social issues. This chapter also shows how nonstandard varieties such as **African American English** and **Chicano English** are rule-governed dialects of English that differ systematically from **Mainstream American English**. This chapter provides suggestions for teachers on how to incorporate sociolinguistic investigations into classroom instruction.

7.2 Dialect

In order to better understand linguistic variation and language in society, it is important to first define some of the key labels for language varieties. One term that is used often but is not well-defined is **dialect**. We have thus far defined language as a human cognitive system that contains the six layers: phonetics, phonology, morphology, syntax, semantics, and pragmatics. If this is what a language is, then what is a dialect? Dialects are sometimes used to describe sub-varieties of a language that are mutually intelligible. Dialects are sometimes used as a term to refer to a deviation from the norm, or something that is spoken by others. Additionally, the word dialect is often used as a diminutive form of language, and as such it is implied that a dialect has limited development, complexity, and usage. A dialect is sometimes used interchangeably with accent or slang. However, these are all myths and misconceptions. Let us explore each one in turn.

The most innocuous of the myths is that dialect is a label for sub-varieties of language, and that dialects are mutually intelligible while languages are not. Mutual intelligibility means that speakers can understand one another's speech variety. It is hypothesized that speakers of different dialects can understand each other but speakers of different languages cannot. However, this is not necessarily true. Mainstream American English speakers, for example, have a difficult time understanding Glaswegian, a variety of Scottish English; not only is the phonology quite different, but the vocabulary and syntactic rules are so different that subtitles or transcripts are often necessary in order to understand the other speaker. If we consider Mainstream American English and Glaswegian dialects of the same language, we would not expect such difficulty with intelligibility. This is the case with the so-called dialects of China as well. Mandarin, Shanghainese, and Cantonese are thought of as dialects of Chinese; however, the three languages are not mutually intelligible. On the other hand, speakers of two separate "languages" can often converse with one another with a fair amount of ease. Spanish and Italian, which are traditionally seen as two different languages, can be mutually intelligible to a limited degree. German and Yiddish are also fairly mutually intelligible, as are Swedish and Norwegian. However, because of political, historical, and social reasons, they are seen as separate languages and not dialects. In sum, we cannot rely on mutual intelligibility as criteria for whether a variety is a language or dialect because there is a significant amount of inconsistency.

Another myth about dialects is that they do not have a fully fledged linguistic system. The implication here is that dialects are less developed and cannot accomplish a full range of purposes. This is not the case. All dialects, whether they have social prestige (Standard American English, Parisian French, Castilian Spanish, Standard Arabic) or are marginalized in society (Chicano English, Senegalese French, Dominican Spanish, Sudanese Arabic), have a full system of phonetics, phonology, morphology, syntax, semantics, and pragmatics. Dominican Spanish, for example, has a regular rule in which /s/ at the end of a syllable becomes /h/: *los manos* → *loh manoh* ("the hands"). This phonological process, called debuccalization, is a common phenomenon across the world's languages, and is a characteristic of Dominican Spanish. Chicano English employs a common grammatical element called null copula, in which the verb *to be* is unnecessary in certain cases: *He funny*. Null copula is employed in other languages such as Russian and American Sign Language. The interesting fact is that when these features appear on "recognized" languages, they get treated as simply a characteristic of the language, but when it appears in low-prestige languages like Dominican Spanish or Chicano English, they are considered evidence of underdevelopment, aberration, or even laziness on the part of the speaker. The fact is, dialects have all the same layers of linguistic complexity as languages, but their treatment in society is unequal.

Related to this, dialects are sometimes thought of as that which is spoken by others, but rarely ourselves. The perception is that dialects are deviations from the norm. The truth is, everybody speaks a dialect. There is no absolute norm in language, the way there is no defined norm in the color of one's skin or the color of one's eyes. As with many facets of society, there is a tendency toward an "us versus them" mentality. To say "we speak a language, but they speak a dialect" might be tempting, but we know there is no way this could be true if everyone said it.

Dialects are sometimes used interchangeably with the term **accent**. The difference, however, is that one's accent is simply the phonetic and phonological patterning. In other words, accent refers to a person's phonetics and phonology layer of their particular language variety. Sometimes, an L2 speaker may sound like they have an accent, and that accent is the phonological patterning of their L1 influencing their L2. However, this is a different concept than dialect. A dialect contains not only just the phonetics and phonology layers, but rather six of the layers we have mentioned before. Figure 7.1 shows the contrast between a dialect and an accent. This is also why it is inaccurate to say that someone does not have an accent or has lost an accent; a person cannot spontaneously lose their phonetics and phonology layers or just not have them. Saying you do not speak with an accent means you have no phonetics or phonology in the way you speak. What people typically mean when they say that someone has an accent is that they do not talk like the so-called norm.

The label dialect also differs from **slang**, which is sometimes used interchangeably with dialect, usually with derogatory or pejorative intent. Slang is used to refer to words or phrases that are relatively new to the language, used in informal settings often to display in-group membership. Sometimes, these slang uses fall out of fashion and are no longer in use: the English word *pickthank* was used in the early 16th century to mean someone who flatters or lies to gain favor. Other times, the slang terminology catches on and becomes widely used, becoming a regular part of the language: the English word *phone* was shortened from *telephone* in the late 19th century when the technology was becoming more widespread. Now, using the word *phone* would not raise

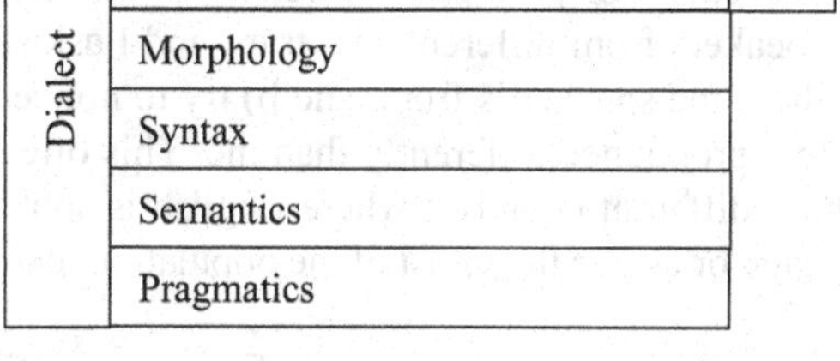

Dialect	Phonetics	Accent
	Phonology	
	Morphology	
	Syntax	
	Semantics	
	Pragmatics	

Figure 7.1 Dialect vs. Accent

any eyebrows or be out of place in formal conversation. In other words, slang only refers to informal fad words, phrases, and expressions of a particular time period, while dialect is a full linguistic system. A dialect can contain slang, but not the other way around. Thus, to call a dialect "slang" would devalue the complexities that a dialect does have.

To circle back to the original question we posed at the beginning of this section, what is the difference between a language and a dialect? We have shown that they are not linguistically different: mutual intelligibility is not accurate criteria, and dialects have a fully fledged grammar just like languages. Dialects are spoken by everyone, and it is distinctly different from an accent or slang. The answer is this: languages and dialects are the same thing. They contain the same layers, have the same level of linguistic complexity, can accomplish multiple purposes, and are governed by rules. The difference between a language and dialect is not a linguistic difference; it's a social difference. Although languages and dialects are equally grammatical and complex, dialects are ones that do not enjoy the same level of prestige. The reason for this can be a number of language external factors. Perhaps the dialect is spoken by groups of people who were historically enslaved or conquered, or by people who are seen as an ethnic minority. Perhaps the dialect is spoken by people who are seen as uneducated or poor or powerless. A language is only recognized as its own language because that variety has garnered importance through being spoken by people who have social and political capital at that time, not because the language itself is particularly special or has superior characteristics. We can call English a dialect, but because of the social power it currently has in our society, it gets elevated to the status of language. As Max Weinreich, a renowned sociolinguist once quipped, "A language is a dialect with an army and a navy".

Voices From the Classroom 7.1—Using TED Talks to Discuss Language Variation

I spend a little bit of time talking about sociolinguistics in my listening classes, because we hear a variety of listening texts, and speakers often have different accents. For example, I have shown different TED talks with English speakers from different countries, and I ask students to a) try to guess where the speaker is from, and b) try to notice three words that the speakers pronounce differently than me. This often opens up a discussion about different countries where English is spoken, either as the main language or as one that most of the population learns in school.

Erica Ashton, ESL Teacher

7.3 Language Variation

One key characteristic of human language is that there is quite a lot of variation. You may have noticed people from other parts of the same country have different words for the same object or concept. There can also be variation even amongst people living in the same geographical region. Two siblings who grew up in the same household may have linguistic differences because their experiences outside of the home differ. People belong to various speech communities, and those speech communities are characterized by a number of sociolinguistic factors. The factors we will discuss next include geography, social class, gender, and age.

7.3.1 Geography

Where you are from and where you live have probably the most obvious impact on your language variety. This makes sense; since language is learned from other people, the people who are in your geographic vicinity can shape your language. A person's geographical location is such a vital part of their language formation that people can sometimes pinpoint where you grew up just from hearing you speak. In fact, you may have seen language surveys online where they ask what you call different items in your dialect, and they can guess what part of the country you grew up in. We know that people speak different languages throughout the world, and even a language that has the same name—English, Arabic, Portuguese—can have marked differences depending on where in the world it is spoken. What is more, even within one country or region, there can be differences at any level of language, whether that be words, pronunciations, or syntax. Let us examine a few of these geographical variants.

A common example of lexical variation by geographical location is *pop-soda-coke*, words that refer to a sweet carbonated beverage, which differ depending on where in the U.S. the word is uttered. In different Spanish-speaking countries, they might use a different word for the same meaning, like *carro* or *coche* for "car" and *jugo* or *zumo* for "juice". In British Sign Language, signs for color words like "brown", "green", and "grey" vary regionally; signers from Belfast, Glasgow, and Newcastle vary in the signing of color words by handshape and/or movement.

Of course, lexical variation is just one small part of language variation. Pronunciation can differ from location to location. In Southern parts of the U.S., the /e/ vowel in English is raised to /i/ before nasal consonants, such that the words *pen* and *pin* or *hem* and *him* are homophonous. Among Spanish-speaking countries, some varieties, such as Castilian Spanish, differentiate between /s/ and /θ/, in which *casa* "house" and *caza* "hunt" are pronounced [kasa] and [kaθa], respectively. In contrast, most of the Spanish spoken in Latin America do not make a distinction between the pronunciation of /s/ and /θ/, and instead both are pronounced as [s], a phenomenon called *seseo*. A third option is *ceceo*, in which both /s/ and /θ/ are pronounced as /θ/. *Ceceo* is employed predominantly in southern parts of Spain.

Voices From the Classroom 7.2—Teaching Dialectal Variation in Spanish Pronunciation

While teaching those language basics to my beginner Spanish 1 class, I made a point to introduce where Spanish is spoken around the world. With that, I explained that different dialects and registers exist in the Spanish language, similar to the English language. We had a whole class discussion about the stereotypes behind different dialects and registers in English. I then connected it to Spanish. The Spanish *ceceo* where the /s/ and /θ/ are pronounced as /θ/ is only spoken in certain parts of the Spanish-speaking world. Some people hold the stereotype that those who use the *ceceo* are speaking "proper" Spanish. However, with hundreds of Spanish language variations exist, it is impossible to gauge which one is "proper" compared to the others. By having this conversation about linguistic variations in Spanish and connecting it to English, students gain new perspectives about their own language as well as the target language being studied.

Isabella Boesso, High School Spanish Teacher

Geographic location can also impact syntactic patterns. In the Southern and Appalachian regions of the U.S., speakers commonly employ double **modals**, a phenomenon in which two (or more) modal auxiliaries are permitted to occur in one clause. Some examples of these can be found in (1) and (2).

(1) She *might could* pick up the groceries.
(2) I *shouldn't oughtta* sleep too late.

Double modal construction is a regular syntactic phenomenon that is widespread across the South and in Appalachian areas, and has become a marker of regional pride and identity. It is used not just in general conversation, but also in literature, politics, and media as a geographic and identity marker. Interestingly, people living in other parts of the country are largely unaware of this syntactic phenomenon.

7.3.2 Social Class

Another variable that has an impact on language is social class. Even if people live in the same geographical area, how they talk can vary depending on the social class they belong to. Although social class does not necessarily determine language, people tend to spend time, socialize, and work with others who are in relatively similar social classes. Because social groups tend to share similar language characteristics, certain linguistic features are associated with social class.

Social class is not an isolated variable, of course. Social class is linked to income, but may not necessarily be interchangeable, as there are high-paying jobs that are associated with working class citizens, and low-paying jobs associated with social prestige. Social class is associated with other social factors such as education and geography, as well as personal factors such as motivation and investment. It is important to note that the varieties of language spoken by people who belong to one social class are not any less developed or complex than those of another social class. However, equally important is how they are perceived by society; historically, people looking to maintain their position in society or be upwardly mobile attempt to shed the linguistic characteristics of the lower social class and adopt the characteristics of the higher social class. We see this in other aspects of society and culture, such as fashion.

One example of linguistic variation linked to social class is the pronunciation of the *-ing* morpheme in English, which is used in progressive participles, gerunds, and adjectives: *He is singing, I enjoy singing, They take singing lessons*. The two most prominent variants for the pronunciation of the *-ing* morpheme are [ɪn] and [ɪŋ], as in *We're workin'* and *We're working*. According to researchers, [ɪn] is used more frequently among lower social classes and [ɪŋ] is used more amongst higher social classes (Labov, 1966; Cofer, 1972; Woods, 1979). Researchers have also found that depending on the formality of context, the same speaker who might use [ɪn] will switch to [ɪŋ], such as in an academic setting. Speakers are more likely to use [ɪŋ] in situations where they may want to showcase their status or education level in society; that same speaker will use [ɪn] in casual, informal contexts.

Another example in which social class plays a role in language is in Montreal French. Poplack and Walker (1986) conducted a study investigating the social factors involved in *l*-deletion, in which /l/ is omitted and sometimes replaced in subject pronouns, object pronouns, and articles. Some examples are *il* "he" [il]→[i] and *elle* "she" [ɛl]→[ɛ]. They found that Montreal French speakers who belong to lower social classes systematically delete /l/ more for all three categories—subject pronouns, object pronouns, and articles—than speakers in higher social classes. This reveals once again that people of different social classes speak differently. Although there is no actual monetary value associated with these arbitrary linguistic features, people begin to associate such features with affluence, power, education, and social capital, however arbitrary the feature might be.

7.3.3 Gender

Language can also vary based on gender. This use of the term gender is different from grammatical gender, which is a system of noun classifications (e.g., masculine, feminine). Here we use gender to refer to that of one's social and personal identity. As gender is very much tied to one's identity, it is thus connected to language and linguistic behavior as well.

Sociolinguists have found that across the world's languages, women tend to speak more of the standard—or most typical—variant of a language than men. For instance, returning to the *-ing* morpheme we discussed previously, women tend to use the [ɪŋ] pronunciation more than men in English. In Labov's study of New York City dialects, findings showed that women tend to use /r/ after a vowel (as in *car* or *circle*) far more frequently than men. Interestingly, we find that when a linguistic innovation—or new phenomenon in language—arises, women are more likely to use that incoming feature than men. For instance, the Northern Cities Chain Shift is a vowel change that is currently ongoing in and around the Great Lakes area of the United States (see Chapter 9 for more information). Eckert (2000) found in her study of adolescent speakers that girls were further along on that chain than boys. In other words, the girls had progressed along the sound change further, and the boys were still behind in that shift.

Another example where gender can impact language variation is from American Sign Language. In parts of the Midwest, the sign for the word "how" in sentence-final position differs between male and female signers. Male-identified signers sign with two A-handshapes and female-identified signers use the Y-handshape for the same meaning. In Figure 7.2 you can see the different handshapes used by the male and female signers to express the same meaning.

One myth associated with language and the role of gender is that women talk more than men. However, research has shown that this is not the case—there is no significant difference between men and women in the number of words they use within the same time frame. What is different is that men tend

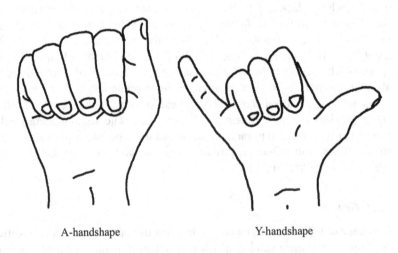

A-handshape   Y-handshape

Figure 7.2 Handshape Variation by Gender in American Sign Language

to spend more time talking than women; put another way, men take up more time in speaking the same amount of words. Consequently, this means women are speaking at a faster rate, which may give the perception that women speak more. Amount of speech is also highly changeable depending on who you are talking to, what you are talking about, and where you are talking. However, there is little evidence that the overall amount of speech differs between men and women.

7.3.4 Age

Another factor that impacts language variation is age. We know that all languages change over time, and it stands to reason that there would be generational differences in how we use and interpret language. You may have heard amusement or discontent from older generations about how language is used by the younger generations. This sort of disgruntlement about language change and language variation by age has been documented throughout history and across the world's languages. This is because linguistic innovations are often brought about by younger people in society, so these new forms might seem different—and are sometimes considered wrong—by older speakers.

An example of age as a factor in language variation is the quotative use of *to be like* in American English. Quotatives are phrases that introduce a quotation, such as *to say* or *to ask*. In the last several decades, the phrasal verb *to be like* has been added to the list of permissible quotatives. Some examples can be seen below:

(3) They were like, "don't ask".
    And then I was like, "why not?"
    And John's like, "trust me".

Studies have shown that the use of quotative *be like* is highly associated with age, such that it is used much more frequently with younger people. For instance, Barbieri (2009) found that speakers above age 40 prefer quotative *say*, while speakers under 40 are more likely to use *be like*. It is quite possible that in another fifty years, the landscape of quotatives will look quite different: for now, there seems to be a generational divide amongst speakers who use and accept *be like* as a quotative.

7.4 Language and Identity

One of the reasons language is so important in our society and to each individual—and why attacks on language are perceived so personally—is that it is intimately linked to one's identity. A person's identity is constructed from a number of factors: age, community, upbringing, education, religion, gender, sexual orientation, media, occupation, ethnicity, socioeconomic status, hobbies or interests. How a person uses and perceives language is constructed by these components as well. The way a person speaks is essentially a manifestation of these facets of identity, and thus being criticized for the way you speak sometimes comes through as a critique of your identity.

Particular lexical items, pronunciation, grammatical patterns, pitch, etc. can be a way that a person marks his or her social identity. Think about how you speak when you are with your closest friends as compared to someone you meet for the first time. Although you are the same person, the vocabulary you choose, the speed at which you talk, and the syntax you use may be very different from one situation to another. These linguistic choices, whether they are conscious or subconscious, are ways you put forth different facets of your identity to suit the situation. One characteristic that many people adopt when in a professional setting is **hypercorrection**, or correcting oneself beyond what is necessary. For example, in schools students are taught to say *and I* in conjoined phrases, such as *my friend and I* or *your mom and I*, instead of *me and my friend* or *me and your mom*. This rule has been drilled so powerfully into our minds that you often hear the *and I* construction as the object of a preposition: *This is for my friend and I* or *Listen to your mom and I*. Technically, the object of a preposition calls for the accusative form of the pronoun (*This is for me* vs. **This is for I*; *Listen to me* vs. **Listen to I*), but because of the explicit teaching in schools, people are prone to hypercorrecting. This small but significant word order signals a certain message. Whether it be "I am educated" or "Please don't think I'm not intelligent" or it is just a force of habit, it reveals something about the speaker's identity. The same with deliberately using the word *pop* in a region where *soda* is prominent, dropping the /r/ in *car*, or using double modals *I might should go*; how a person speaks is a (not so) subtle realization of their social identity.

Relatedly, language can be a marker of in-group membership, a linguistic badge that indicates belongingness to a **speech community**. Think about a community that you belong to—whether that be sports, hobbies, or occupation—and the specialized vocabulary you use with others in that community. Do you use words or phrases within this group that might not make any sense to outsiders? This is what linguists call **jargon**, or specialized vocabulary for a particular interest group. Jargon is often used to signal this in-group membership. For instance, in the field of education, one might use abbreviations such as *IEP*, *EL*, and *SPED* that people outside of the field might not be familiar with. Musicians have their own set of jargon, such as *coda* (the end tag of a musical number), *the top* (the beginning), *key change* (modulation of the tonic), and *legato* (play connectedly). Knitting communities have words like *cast on* (to start a new project), *to frog* (to unravel), *k2tog* (knit two stitches together), and *hank* (unwound twisted bundle of yarn). Sports, hobbies, occupations, and other special-interest communities often have their own set of jargon that is not only helpful to talk about the topics amongst themselves but demonstrate in-group membership and community. In other words, the jargon is useful not only as a shorthand amongst in-group members, but also as a linguistic indicator that you are part of the community and "in the know".

Another example of language as a marker of community is the way code-switching is used in bilingual communities. Code-switching is the phenomenon in which two or more languages are used within speech (see also Chapter 10). Bilingual speakers, children and adults alike, often code-switch with other bilingual speakers to show closeness, respect, community, and belongingness. There are two important things to note about code-switching. Firstly, code-switching is used only with other people who speak the same languages. Rarely will you find an example in which a Spanish-English bilingual will code-switch with a monolingual English speaker. This is because bilingual speakers are keenly aware of who is part of their community, as well as the language preferences of their interlocutors. Secondly, code-switching has regular rules, just like dialects. For instance, one cannot simply switch from language A to language B every other word. There are grammatical rules as to where switches can and cannot occur. Both of these facts—that code-switching is used with other bilinguals and has rules—indicate that it is not an indication of confusion or lack of proficiency; in fact, code-switching requires proficiency of the two languages to switch seamlessly between the two languages. Switching between two languages signals to the bilingual interlocutor that you are both part of the same community, whether it be of immigrants, heritage language speakers, or learners of a second language.

Dialects are often used as an indicator of one's in-group membership. African American English (AAE), for instance, is not just a system of complex syntax, phonology, semantics, etc., but a signal of one's heritage, culture, and community. Many African American in the U.S., for instance, use AAE with other members of the community as a symbol of pride, belongingness, and closeness. Although certain features of AAE have been negatively targeted in mainstream U.S., members of AAE-speaking communities have reclaimed these features as an integral part of their linguistic and cultural identity. This is what is known as covert prestige, or high value placed on a nonstandard variety. We will explore some of these features later in the chapter.

7.5 Language and Discrimination

Thus far, we have seen how languages vary based on a number of factors, and that language is an integral part of one's identity. If this were the extent of it, the world would be a happy place. However, it is perhaps because of these facts—that everyone speaks differently and that language is a marker of identity—that language sometimes becomes a tool for discrimination.

Think of a time when you have been scolded or laughed at because of the way you talk. Perhaps someone has pointed out to you that you say a word funny or wrong. Or maybe you have witnessed this happening to someone you know. On a small scale, noticing differences in the way we talk can be fun and eye-opening. But because there are so many factors associated with language—geography, social class, gender, age, as well as the multiple facets of one's identity—it can be a source of discriminatory practice. Making fun of how someone pronounces a word is not simply a comment on the vowel they choose; it is a comment on their background or where they come from. Telling a heritage language speaker that their grammar is incorrect is not simply a comment on their syntax; it is a comment on their families who raised them. Because language is a reflection of one's identity, ridiculing or threatening their language can be a veiled attack on their identity.

Interestingly, people can get away with making statements about someone's language much more easily than they can about someone's race, ethnicity, or religion. Imagine a scenario where a teacher says aloud in class "the color of your skin is wrong; let me show you how you can correct it" or "your religious beliefs are wrong; let me show you the right one". Such a blatant disrespect for something that is an integral part of a student's identity might make you uncomfortable. However, it is not uncommon to hear a teacher say, "the way you speak is wrong; let me show you how you can correct it". This is a trickier nuance, because a language teacher's job is to teach language. However, there is a difference between "wrong" and "different", even in language. Some features are perceived as being wrong, even though that feature is simply a characteristic within that language or dialect. For instance, it is considered "wrong" to end a sentence with a preposition:

(4)   Who did you go with?
(5)   What did you do that for?

But if you look at how often people end sentences with prepositions, you will find that it occurs quite frequently. In fact, in regular conversation it sounds rather awkward and stilted to change the structure so that it does not end in a preposition: *With whom did you go?* or *For what did you do that?*

Examples like these are easier to digest and easier to teach because most majority language speakers will agree that while you are supposed to say it one way, the reality is that no one really talks like that. But when the targeted features are spoken predominantly by speakers that are otherwise marginalized or disadvantaged in society, it becomes trickier to discern. Let us consider three such examples.

Double negatives are a phenomenon in which there are two or more negation words—or **negative polarity items** (NPIs)—with a negative value in a clause. Some NPIs with a negative value are *not, neither, never, no, none, nowhere, no one, nobody*. An example of a clause with more than two or more negative value NPIs are below:

(6)   I do<u>n't</u> have <u>none</u>.
(7)   I <u>never</u> go <u>nowhere</u>.
(8)   There's <u>no</u> one here <u>neither</u>

Languages that utilize this grammatical feature are known as having **negative concord**, in which two negative words still equal a negative meaning. Languages that have negative concord include Spanish, Portuguese, Polish, Hebrew, Ukrainian, and Russian. African American English and Chicano English also have negative concord. However, **Mainstream American English** (MAE) is a language that does not have negative concord anymore[1]. In MAE, if there is a negative value NPI in the clause, then the other NPIs in the clause must have positive value. Some examples of NPIs with positive value are *any, anyone, anywhere, anyway, either, even, ever*. Thus, in dialects of MAE, it is typical that speakers will say "I don't have any", "I never go anywhere", and "there's no one here either" instead of the versions in (6) through (8). Other languages that do not have negative concord include German and Dutch.

If we view this simply as a linguistic difference—some languages have this feature, other languages do not have this feature—it would not be much of a problem. However, because many English speakers do not realize and recognize that African American English or Chicano English are fully fledged languages with their own grammatical systems, speakers of MAE mistakenly believe that there is something wrong with using two NPIs within the same clause. Instead of realizing that this is a grammatical difference between two dialects, teachers will often correct the student who is utilizing negative concord. Often, the implication of using double negatives is that the student is confused or has issues with logic ("in math, two negatives make a positive!"). This happens often with minority language speakers. However, rarely does anyone comment that all Russian or Spanish speakers—speakers who systematically use negative concord in their languages—are confused or have issues with logic. Because of the status of the speakers who use negative concord in the U.S., this particular feature becomes targeted.

Another linguistic feature that is targeted as a result of its speakers is **upspeak** and **vocal fry**. Upspeak, also known as uptalk, is a phenomenon in which declarative sentences end with a rising intonation. Vocal fry, or creaky voice, is almost the opposite, in which the speaker uses a deep, creaky tone of voice that is made by relaxing the vocal cords but expelling the same amount of air, resulting in a creaky tone. Both upspeak and vocal fry are generally associated with young female speakers. The general criticism underlying upspeak is that declarative sentences are supposed to have falling intonation, and that ending them with a rising intonation makes them sound like questions. However, the reality is that questions in English usually have falling intonation. For example, wh-questions in English have falling intonation, as in (9) and (10). Tag questions that are used to request confirmation also have falling intonation, as in (11) and (12).

(9)   What are you ⟍doing?
(10) How did you know ⟍that?
(11) That's yours, isn't ⟍it?
(12) I'm in your way, aren't ⟍I?

Women are often criticized for using upspeak because it allegedly demonstrates nonassertive and submissive behavior. However, men also use upspeak quite regularly (Ritchart & Arvaniti, 2014; Levon, 2016; Prechtel, 2015), but this behavior in men is not seen as unassertive or submissive, but rather polite and considerate (Linneman, 2013).

Similarly, vocal fry is seen as a negative stereotype of young women, and that when used, it supposedly makes them seem less competent, less educated, and less hirable (Anderson, Klofstad, Mayew, & Venkatachalam, 2014). Of course, this is arbitrary, as changing one's vocal cord laxness obviously does not affect one's abilities or education level. Vocal fry is actually utilized in languages as a phonemic contrast: for example, in Danish, a word pronounced with creaky voice and without creaky voice have two different meanings, forming a minimal pair. The word *løber* with creaky voice means "run (verb)" and *løber* without creaky voice means "runner". Here is yet another example of linguistic features that are used as a proxy or scapegoat for underlying societal inequities. By pointing out an arbitrary linguistic feature as the reason for maltreatment or unfairness, it places the burden of inequity on the already marginalized group of people. While it is not well received to say "you are not going to be taken seriously because you are a young woman", it is somehow perfectly acceptable to say "you are not going to be taken seriously because you use vocal fry". The takeaway is not that young women should stop using upspeak or vocal fry; it is that societally, we take these arbitrary linguistic features to further marginalize young women.

Finally, another feature that gets negative attention is r-lessness, a phenomenon in which the /r/ sound is dropped at ends of words and syllables. This is typically found in the Boston area or parts of New York City, where *car, four*, and *butter* might sound like *cah, foh*, and *buttah*. Media portrayals of speakers of r-lessness propagates the stereotype that the speakers are uneducated, unintelligent, and rude, and are associated with working class, low income individuals. What is interesting is that this same phenomenon of r-lessness is seen as a desirable characteristic if it is used by a British English speaker. British English speakers are generally seen as sophisticated, posh, and intelligent by many American English speakers. The double standard is rather striking; if the /r/ is dropped by a Bostonian or New Yorker, it is an indication of lack of education and low income, and if the /r/ is dropped by a Londoner, it is a marker of refinement. Once again, our society has linked a random aspect of language with judgment about the people who speak it.

These examples—double negatives, upspeak, vocal fry, and r-lessness—are linguistically neutral features that appear frequently across the world's languages or are common phenomena that expand beyond just the targeted group. However, they are arbitrarily and disproportionately used to demean groups of speakers that are already marginalized in society. As we discussed, it is not acceptable to openly degrade a person due to their race, ethnicity, or gender; however, it is unfortunately common practice to degrade a person's language. This extends in the classroom as well: students who speak a nonstandard variety of a language are sometimes not seen for what they are—speakers of another dialect—but instead are treated as if they learned the language wrong. The key is this: languages and dialects are linguistically equal but socially unequal. If you look at the speakers that are negatively targeted for using double negatives, upspeak, vocal fry, and r-lessness, you will notice one common factor: they are already disadvantaged in some way, whether it be due to race, ethnicity, age, gender, or socioeconomic status. The linguistic feature that receives the negative attention is often used to explain away why the speaker is disadvantaged, with promises such as "you will get a better job if you stop X" or "people will take you more seriously if you Y". Of course, if a single consonant or use of a different NPI could magically change one's outcome such that they would no longer be subject to discrimination, our society would be perfect now. What happens after a young woman decides to stop using upspeak? What happens after an African American English speaker stops using negative concord? Does that eliminate sexism, ageism, or racism?

7.6 Nonstandard Dialects

So far we talked about how languages and dialects are used as a tool for discrimination, and specific features are further used as a scapegoat for marginalization of a group or community. When this is done on an even larger scale in which entire dialects—not just single consonants or grammatical rules—are targeted, these are often referred to as **nonstandard dialects**.

Before moving forward, let us consider this idea of a standard versus a nonstandard dialect. A **standard dialect** is often thought of as the agreed-upon variety of a language that is used across an area. While this can be true in some places where a governing body makes decisions on what the standard variety looks and sounds like, there are some incorrect assumptions made about standard varieties that do not hold true. For one, the general public largely assumes that the standard variety is the correct version and nonstandard varieties are incorrect deviations from the norm. This is not true: all dialects (whether standard or nonstandard, powerful or not) are just as correct, logical, developed, and rule based as any other dialect or language in the world. Again, the difference between a standard dialect and a nonstandard dialect is that the standard variety has societal recognition, power, and authority, none of which has anything to do with the linguistic characteristics of that dialect. However, because of that power and recognition, the so-called standard variety is seen as official and authoritative.

The second faulty assumption is that the standard dialect is unchanging and fixed. This is not true because all languages change over time, and the only time a language does not change is when there are no speakers left. If you listen to a television news broadcast from today, then from ten years ago and from fifty years ago, you will likely hear a difference in the way that the broadcaster speaks. The third fallacy is that standard languages do not vary from speaker to speaker and from place to place. However, even within one country that claims to speak the same standard language, there will be differences at all levels of language: phonetics, phonology, morphology, syntax, and so on. A broadcaster speaking standard American English in California will sound different from a broadcaster speaking standard American English in Kansas. A speaker using standard Italian in Milan will have distinct differences from a speaker using standard Italian in Naples. Variation is a key trait in all human language, and standard languages are not exempt from that characteristic.

What is the difference between a standard and nonstandard dialect, then? Again, this goes back to our previous discussion on the difference between a language and a dialect. The only difference is that a standard dialect is often dubbed a language and is the variety that holds and represents social capital, while the nonstandard dialect is linguistically every bit as equal as the standard variety but lacks overt social prestige and status.

7.6.1 African American English

One prominent nonstandard dialect in the U.S. is African American English (AAE). Earlier in this chapter, we talked about how AAE is a proud marker of heritage, culture, and community and carries covert prestige. Linguistically, AAE is a fully fledged language with its own system of phonetics, phonology, morphology, syntax, semantics, and pragmatics. AAE has within it multiple registers, as well as regional, socioeconomic, gender, and generational variation. There are a number of linguistic characteristics that are common amongst most varieties of AAE and we will cover a few of these in what follows; however, it is important to note that not all AAE looks, sounds, or works the same way.

A phonological characteristic of AAE is **consonant cluster reduction**. This is a phenomenon in which word-final consonant blends such as /sk/, /st/, /nd/ and /ld/ are simplified to a single consonant. Some examples can be seen in Table 7.1 below.

This is neither an aberration or cause for concern. In fact, consonant cluster reduction is seen across the world's languages. Historically, Mainstream English speakers used to pronounce the -*ng* consonant cluster as [ng], but over time this has reduced to one consonant, [ŋ]. Many of the world's languages, such as Hawaiian, Japanese, and Finnish, do not permit consonant clusters in word-final position. AAE is simply another language of the world that has this consonant cluster restriction as a regular phonological rule.

Table 7.1 Contrast Between Mainstream and African American English

Mainstream American English	African American English
Task	Tas
Test	Tes
Sand	San
Cold	Col

Another linguistic characteristic of AAE is that it allows the copula to be dropped in some grammatical cases, a phenomenon called **null copula** or **zero copula**. A copula is a verb (such as the verb *to be*) that links the subject and the predicate. Some examples of copula deletion can be seen in (13) below.

(13) a. Dee is the choir director. vs. Dee ø the choir director.
     b. Dee is nice. vs. Dee ø nice.
     c. Dee is in the library. vs. Dee ø in the library.

             (Green, 2002, p. 684)

Although many MAE speakers believe AAE null copula is done randomly, there are strict rules that apply. Firstly, null copula is only allowed when the verb is in the present tense. Secondly, the subject must be third person. Thirdly, null copula is never allowed at the end of a sentence (*I don't know who he is* vs. **I don't know who he ø*) nor in a tag question (*That's not him, is it?* vs. **That's not him, ø it?*). Null copula is a well-documented phenomenon across many of the world's languages, including Russian, Turkish, American Sign Language, Hungarian, and Ganda; however, AAE speakers who use this grammatical rule and do omit the copula in these specialized cases are seen as using English with incorrect grammar. This view stems from a misunderstanding of the rules of AAE, and more broadly speaking, failure to realize that AAE is a separate language with its own separate grammatical rules.

The last feature of AAE that we will discuss is the use of habitual *be*. In some languages, there is a morphological distinction between actions that are one-time occurrences and actions that are ongoing and habitual. French and Spanish make this distinction between past tense verbs: the verb will change endings depending on whether the action in the past was a one-time completed action versus an ongoing habitual action. MAE speakers have difficulty with this because MAE makes no such distinction. In MAE, the sentence *I rode the bus to school* can mean either (a) the speaker rode the bus to school that one particular time, or that (b) the speaker regularly rode the bus to school as the mode of transportation. In AAE, however, the language makes the distinction with habitual *be*. Habitual *be* is an aspectual marker that signals that the action was done on a regular basis, and always appears in the infinitive form.

(14) a. Dee be running. "Dee is usually running" or "Dee usually runs"
     b. Dee IS running. "Dee is running now"
     c. Dee ø running. "Dee is running now"

             (Green, 2002, p. 682)

In (14a), the aspectual marker *be* indicates that the action of running is a habitual action. In contrast, if the speaker conjugates the verb *to be*, as in (14b), or drops it altogether, as in (14c), the new interpretation of the sentence is that the subject is running right now. Because the aspect is encoded in the auxiliary, AAE speakers do not have to use adverbial phrases like *now* or *usually*, making it arguably more efficient than MAE. This is difficult for MAE speakers to interpret. Teachers unfamiliar with AAE will often interpret all three sentences in (14) as having the same meaning, assuming that the student cannot conjugate the verb *to be* or is using the verb randomly. The misunderstanding of the dialectal difference can lead to wrongful classification of the student as having a speech or learning problem. Thus, it is important for teachers to understand some of the features of nonstandard dialects like AAE in order to better serve linguistically diverse students.

7.6.2 Chicano English

Chicano English (ChE) is a variety of English spoken primarily by Mexican Americans in the U.S. Like AAE, ChE is a fully fledged language with its own set of rules and characteristics. ChE is also a language variety that carries a great amount of covert prestige and is a cultural asset and marker of identity for many individuals of Mexican descent. However, because ChE is associated with a marginalized population within the U.S., the language also receives negative attention. Much of the misunderstanding behind ChE stems from its lack of recognition as a language. It is mistakenly believed to be poorly spoken English, incorrect Spanish, or learner language (a Spanish speaker who speaks English as a second language). ChE is none of those things; it is an established language that has all the layers of language we have discussed. ChE speakers are often bilingual in ChE and MAE and can switch back and forth between the two languages. ChE can be learned as a child's first language, and a person can be a monolingual speaker of ChE, just as one can be a monolingual speaker of Arabic, Cantonese, or Mainstream American English.

One feature of ChE is /z/ devoicing, in which the voiced alveolar fricative is changed to a voiceless alveolar fricative, /s/. Similarly, the voiced labiodental fricative /v/ is devoiced to /f/ in word final position. Some examples of devoicing in ChE are seen in Table 7.2.

Devoicing of voiced consonants is a common phonological process across the world's languages. In German and Polish, for example, consonants that appear at the ends of words are devoiced. In many varieties of English, word final **obstruents** are voiced when pluralized but devoiced in the singular, such as *knife-knives* [naif]-[nai<u>vz</u>] and *mouth-mouths* [mɑʊθ]-[mɑʊ<u>ð</u>z].

Table 7.2 Devoicing in Chicano English

Word	Mainstream American English pronunciation	Chicano English pronunciation
Zero	[ziroʊ]	[siroʊ]
Busy	[bɪzi]	[bɪsi]
Size	[saɪz]	[saɪs]
Save	[seiv]	[seif]
Lives	[laivz]	[laifs]

Table 7.3 Verb Paradigm in Mainstream American English

	Singular	Plural
1st person	I play	We play
2nd person	You play	You (y'all, you guys) play
3rd person	He/she/it plays	They play

ChE is another language that allows negative concord, or double negatives. In ChE, multiple NPIs are allowed to be used within one clause, and the resulting meaning is still negative, such as in *They didn't see nothing* or *He won't talk to no one.* Again, this is a feature of many languages throughout the world.

Another feature of ChE is that it regularizes verb conjugations. In MAE, the third person singular conjugation is the only form of the verb that is different, as you can see from Table 7.3.

In ChE, however, the irregular conjugation for third person singular is regularized, a process called **paradigm leveling**. Thus, the paradigm for ChE would utilize *play* for all persons and numbers: *I play, you play, he/she/it play, we play, you play, they play.* Regularization of irregular forms and paradigm leveling are common processes across the world's languages. It also has had a major impact on what we know as English today (see Chapter 9 for more information). However, what is interesting is that this regularization is seen as a natural historical process when it happens to languages of power but is seen as incorrect grammar or an aberration when it occurs in nonstandard languages. Once again, it is important for teachers to keep in mind that difference does not equate incorrectness when it comes to dialectal differences.

7.7 Incorporating Sociolinguistics in the Language Classroom

As we have learned this chapter, how one speaks is a marker of identity, and by affirming students' home languages, we affirm their identities. In order for teachers to support linguistic diversity among their students, it must begin with teachers' own evaluation of their ideologies. One exercise that teachers can do is to think about all the different registers, dialects, and languages we speak. Even if you may consider yourself monolingual, you might realize that you speak in many different ways depending on the group or person you're speaking with, the context, the topic, or even your mood. You can explore this further in the exercises section at the end of this chapter.

It is also important for students learning a second language to know that even though the textbook might prescribe just one standard, homogenous target language, the reality is that people speak differently. Teachers can find video or audio clips of speakers of the target language from different areas of the world or country and play these for the learners. Then, ask students to identify differences between the varieties. In addition to these regional variations, students are often interested to learn that within the target language, real speakers use slang, abbreviations, and other registers. Allow students to explore how young people who speak the target language use certain linguistic features that are of informal register, like texting. We often sterilize the target language in our effort to make it easier to learn, but we forget that the real language "in the wild" is diverse and relatable to our students. Tapping into this can be a great lesson and motivator.

For **heritage language learners**, the goal of affirming students' linguistic identities is even more critical. Heritage language learners may speak the target language at home, but may not have developed literacy skills or academic vocabulary and grammar in their heritage language since there is usually little need for these skills in a home setting. Additionally, heritage language learners often speak low prestige or marginalized varieties of the language. When heritage language learners take their own language as a subject at school, their languages are sometimes met with rejection. They may be told that their home variety is not the "standard", or that their vocabulary or grammar is wrong. They may be told that they don't write well, and that they have been speaking wrong all their lives. Since students' identities are intricately linked to their home language, this rejection of their home language variety becomes a rejection of their identities, as well as their families and heritage. One way to affirm the identities and languages of heritage language learners is to first adopt the attitude that their linguistic variety is valid and correct. Together with a class, make a list of all the ways to say the same thing, regardless of whether it is formal or informal, delicate or blunt. There tends to be a lot of variation amongst languages and dialects when it comes to idiomatic expressions, especially for taboo topics, so that is a fun place to start. Heritage students can be a wealth of information when it comes to these types of linguistic expressions.

Bilingual classrooms are set up perfectly for comparison and evaluation of linguistic variation. Because there is already an established multilingual context, students in these settings are already adept at noticing differences between languages. Teachers sometimes remark, however, that one language tends to have a higher status among students, an attitude which can sometimes come from the rest of the school, other teachers, or other students in the school. Students can explore this: although we typically think of the classroom as being bilingual, each of the two languages has a lot of variation and complexity. For instance, in a Spanish-English dual language classroom, students can brainstorm all the different dialects of Spanish they can come up with, and what characterizes each one. They can also generate the many different levels of formality one can use in Spanish. Then, repeat the same exercise in English. By doing this, students can see that both languages have these variations and complexities, and both languages are used widely and by many people in different ways and different settings.

Voices From the Classroom 7.3—Linguistic Variation in a Dual Language Classroom Setting

S1: Teacher, I just finished coloring my *chuchito*.
T: What does that word mean?
S2: *Chuchito* is the way you say dog in Guatemala.
T: Thank you for teaching me a new word. Let's add it to our Regionalisms chart!

This scenario is common in my third grade classroom. Linguistic variation refers to the regional, social, or contextual differences in the ways that a particular language is used. In my classroom I have newcomer students from Mexico and Guatemala, as well as students who have grown up in the U.S. A goal of dual language education is to help students develop socio cultural competence. Students should be able to see the similarities and differences in each other, but view the differences as opportunities to connect rather than as obstacles to overcome. In order to capture and celebrate the linguistic variety in my classroom, I have created a Regionalisms anchor chart where we add words that are said differently in different countries. Our conversations around language variation have enriched and expanded my students' linguistic repertoires and have helped to create a learning environment that celebrates linguistic diversity.

Érik Martínez, Third Grade Bilingual Teacher

Another way to incorporate sociolinguistics in the language classroom is to have the students conduct sociolinguistic experiments of their own. In an ESL class, for instance, groups of students can conduct a study of linguistic variation among English speakers by interviewing native speakers, having them read something, or even eliciting certain responses. A chance to collect actual data can be an engaging exercise for students, not only to learn about language variation, but also to conduct research of their own on the very language they are studying.

Further Reading

Fought, C. (2003). *Chicano English in context*. London: Palgrave Macmillan.

Lippi-Green, R. (2012). *English with an accent: Language, ideology, and discrimination in the United States* (2nd ed.). New York: Routledge.

McWhorter, J. H. (2017). *Talking back, talking Black: Truths about America's Lingua Franca*. New York: Bellevue Literary Press.

Meyerhoff, M. (2018). *Introducing sociolinguistics* (3rd ed.). New York: Routledge.

Exercises

1. Find an animated children's movie and identify the main and supporting characters. Listen to the voices of each character and the dialect used for that character. Consider the questions below:

   a. How does the dialect or accent contribute to the character's persona?
   b. Are there any stereotypes being propagated about the dialect?

2. Create a dialect survey by coming up with a few pictures of objects that might be called different things in the target language. Ask as many people as you can to get their responses, and ask them a few biographical questions, like where they grew up, their age, gender, etc. Collect the responses to see if any patterns arise based on any of the biographical information.

3. People use different registers, or levels of formality, depending on the situation. Compare how you would convey the following messages in a formal email versus an informal text message. How does the language differ?

   a. Cancel an appointment that is happening one hour from now.
   b. Express thanks for a gift.
   c. Tell them good personal news.

4. Make a list of two or three different languages, dialects, or registers you use on a regular basis, and see if you can identify what role each of those varieties play in your life. Describe when and where you use each of these varieties, and how you see yourself when speaking these varieties. Do you make efforts to shape your language to fit the expectations of your circumstances, or do you consciously oppose these expectations through your language use? Think about any feelings of pride, shame, belongingness, alienation, and professionalism that characterize each of those varieties. Analyzing your own language use and linguistic identities may help you realize that your students experience these as well.

Note

1. Historically, Mainstream American English did have negative concord, but lost it sometime around the 16th and 17th centuries.

References

Anderson, R. C., Klofstad, C. A., Mayew, W. J., & Venkatachalam, M. (2014). Vocal fry may undermine the success of young women in the labor market. *PLoS One, 9*(5).

Barbieri, F. (2009). Quotative be like in American English: Ephemeral or here to stay? *English World-Wide, 30*, 68–90.

Cofer, T. (1972). *Linguistic variability in a Philadelphia community* (dissertation). University of Pennsylvania, Philadelphia.

Eckert, P. (2000). *Language variation as social practice: The linguistic construction of identity in belten high.* Hoboken, NJ: Wiley.

Green, L. (2002). A descriptive study of African American English: Research in linguistics and education. *International Journal of Qualitative Studies in Education, 15*(6), 673–690. https://doi.org/10.1080/0951839022000014376

Labov, W. (1966). *The social stratification of English in New York City.* Washington, DC: Center for Applied Linguistics.

Levon, E. (2016). Gender, interaction and intonational variation: The discourse functions of high rising terminals in London. *Journal of Sociolinguistics, 20*(2), 133–163.

Linneman, T. J. (2013). Gender in jeopardy! Intonation variation on a television game show. *Gender & Society, 27*(1), 82–105.

Poplack, S., & Walker, D. (1986). Going through (L) in Canadian French. In D. Sankoff (Ed.), *Diversity and diachrony* (pp. 173–198). https://doi.org/10.1075/cilt.53.17pop

Prechtel, C. (2015). *Effects of gender and regional dialect on uptalk in the American Midwest* (Unpublished BA dissertation). The Ohio State University, Columbus, OH.

Ritchart, A., & Arvaniti, A. (2014). The form and use of uptalk in southern Californian English. In *Proceedings of the international conference on speech prosody* (pp. 331–336). Dublin, Ireland: Trinity College Dublin.

Woods, H. (1979). *A socio-dialectal survey of the English spoken in Ottawa: A study of sociolinguistic and stylistic variation* (dissertation). University of Ottawa, Ottawa.

8   Languages in Contact

8.1 Introduction

The world we live in is constantly changing, and language comes along for that ride, being shaped by that change. Language contact occurs when speakers of two or more varieties meet, interact, and influence one another. What are ways that languages come into contact, and what happens when they do? Much in the way that two colors of paint mix, swirl, and blend, creating something new, languages react and change when they come into prolonged contact with one another. In this chapter, we describe how pidgins develop and the ways in which these rudimentary contact varieties are used for communication despite their limited vocabularies and grammars. We also explain how the vocabulary and grammar of pidgins undergo expansion through creolization. This chapter describes properties of some of the localized varieties of English that have developed in different areas of the world, and the role of English as a lingua franca in the contemporary world.

8.2 Contact Situations

Before we talk about what happens to languages when they come into contact, it is worthwhile to explore how languages come into contact in the first place. In what situations do two or more languages end up in the same place at the same time? Travel, certainly, is one way we are exposed to new languages—many people use apps or books to learn the target language before traveling to a new country. Relatedly, geographic proximity is another way two languages might come into contact. Perhaps even more relevant for us is that language contact often occurs in education, in the form of taking a second or foreign language as a subject, or being taught other content in a language different than the one you speak at home. Languages also come into contact when people move to a new place, as in migration. In fact, many of the languages in the Americas were brought over from other places in the world. Business and trade can also lead to language contact. When two different communities need resources that can be supplied by the other community, the two groups have to come into contact to conduct business.

Technology also plays a significant role in language contact. When travel, exploration, and migration became facilitated by ships, trains, automobiles, and later air travel, distant societies that had never had the opportunity to come into contact did so more easily and more frequently. If previously a geographical barrier existed, such as a mountain or ocean, technology allowed people to dig through, surmount, or cross over the barrier and come into contact with new societies. More recently, information technology has revolutionized the way human societies communicate with one another. With the rise of the internet, one can instantaneously reach someone on the other side of the world, find information about a language or culture, and listen to music sung in hundreds of languages. Language teachers can easily find videos of the target language and share it with the class, an option that became available only relatively recently. With the advent of information technology, the languages and cultures of people living in faraway places come right into our classrooms and handheld devices.

Unfortunately, language contact is not always as peaceful and benevolent as the foregoing examples. In fact, a great deal of language contact is the result of violent, unjust, harrowing experiences such as war, conquest, occupation, and slavery. The history of human civilization is riddled with examples in which one group of people decides to dominate, enslave, forcibly remove, or kill another group of people in the interest of some gain. In these cases of language contact, there is often a clear language of power, held by those in the dominant position, and a language of the oppressed, held by the subjugated peoples. However, as we will discuss in this chapter, even in these violent language contact situations, the natural path of language change carries on, and new forms of communication and new languages are born from these events in history.

8.3 Borrowing

What happens when languages come into contact with one another? A common phenomenon that occurs is **borrowing**, in which an element of one language is permanently added to the linguistic repertoire of another language. This can be at the lexical, phonetic, phonological, morphological, syntactic, semantic, or pragmatic levels. One only has to flip through an English dictionary and note the etymology of words in the English language to see how most words originate from some other language, including Latin, Greek, French, Arabic, and German. Borrowing is different from code-switching in that borrowing results in a linguistic element that permanently embeds itself into the borrowing language, taking on the features of the borrowing language. Monolingual speakers still use borrowed features without having any competence in the source language, e.g., most English speakers use plenty of French-origin words without actually speaking French. In contrast, code-switching is the alternating use of two or more languages within a conversation. It is done by bilinguals when they are in the company of other bilinguals. You have to be bilingual in order to code-switch.

Borrowing does not mean that the borrowed word, sound, or grammar rule is preserved perfectly in its original form. Much like the way a liquid poured from one container into another will take the form of that new container, the borrowed element may still resemble the original characteristics, but it will also conform to the established rules of the borrowing language. In the following we will explore examples of lexical and structural borrowing, and how that borrowed element changes its shape, as well as how that borrowed element changes the shape of the borrowing language.

8.3.1 Lexical Borrowing

Perhaps the most easily identified borrowing is **lexical borrowing**, in which words and phrases are borrowed from one language to another. Lexical borrowing happens very frequently in a vast array of contexts. Words pertaining to foods are a common example, where it is simply easiest to just use the native word for the food item; *kimchi, tortilla, sushi, biscotti, hummus, bratwurst, naan,* and *borscht* are much easier—and sound more appetizing—than spicy fermented cabbage or flat-pressed disk of corn or flour. Terms referring to technology are often borrowed from English into other languages, especially in areas with frequent English contact. Words like *email, wifi,* and *to print* are borrowed into Spanish as *el email, el wifi,* and *printear.* Words and phrases in English that pertain to academia and theater are often Greek in origin: *grammar, physics, chorus, monologue, protagonist.* Many of the words we use regularly in English also originate from Native American languages, like *chocolate* (Nahuatl: *chocolatl*), *chipmunk* (Ojibwa: *chitmunk*), *squash* (Narragansett: *askútasquash*), *barbecue* (Taíno: *barbacòa*), *moose* (Eastern Abenaki: *moz*), *kayak* (Inuktitut: *qajaq*). If you look up word origins in your native or target language, you may unearth some surprising origin stories for words you have always thought of as mundane.

What is perhaps even more interesting is what happens when that word or phrase is borrowed. Think about the word *taco,* and how it is pronounced in mainstream American English. The /t/ and /k/ sounds are probably both aspirated, like the /t/ in the word *top* or the /k/ in the word *coat.* The /o/ is likely to be a diphthong, sounding more like [ow], like we discussed in Chapter 2. However, if you hear or say the word *taco* in the lender language of Spanish, the /t/ and /k/ are unaspirated like in *stop* or *score,* and the /o/ is a pure vowel [o]. In fact, some Spanish-speakers have a hard time understanding the English-speaker's pronunciation of words borrowed from Spanish because the pronunciation is very different. This does not have anything to do with malintent; the borrowed word just has to change to fit the **phonotactic rules** of the borrowing language.

English words that are borrowed into other languages have to go through the same process as well. The words *printear* ("to print") and *parquear* ("to park") have been borrowed from English by Spanish-speakers in the U.S., even though there are Spanish equivalents for the word already: *imprimir* and *estacionar*, respectively. The reason for this is most likely geographical proximity, as languages that are in physical contact have an obvious reason and opportunity for influencing one another, a natural occurrence. But, because Spanish has a full-fledged paradigm of conjugation based on infinitive verbs that end with *-ar, -er*, or *-ir*, the verbs *print* and *park* were converted to have an ending that makes it easy to then conjugate for person and number. Another example comes from the various ways that other languages have adopted the greeting *Merry Christmas*. In Japanese, a language that does not allow many consonant clusters or syllable-final consonants, the phrase becomes *Meri Kurisumasu*. Similarly, in Maori it becomes *Meri Kirihimete*. In Hawaiian, which also has strict rules about consonant clusters and additionally does not employ the /r/ sound at all, the phrase becomes *Mele Kalikimaka*, made popular in a cheery song.

8.3.2 Structural Borrowing

Sometimes, when a language borrows enough words from another language, entire structures that did not originally exist in the borrowing language end up becoming a permanent feature. This is called **structural borrowing**. For instance, at the phonetics and phonology levels, sounds or sound patterns that did not exist before can be added to the phonetic inventory or system of phonological rules. For instance, the /ʒ/ sound that you find in words like *measure, treasury, siege, beige*, and *mirage* did not exist in the English phonetic inventory until its contact with French. But through continuous contact with French, the /ʒ/ became part of English. In Spanish, velar fricatives /x/ and /ɣ/ in words like *reloj* [relox] ("clock") and *jugo* [xuɣo] ("juice") did not exist in the language until its extensive contact with Arabic.

When words are borrowed from one language to another, the morphological process that goes along with the source language can be borrowed as well. For instance, some pluralization rules in English originate from languages like Latin and Greek. Instead of regular pluralization where /s/, /z/, and /ɪz/ are added, some words take on irregular endings when a singular noun becomes plural. Some examples from Latin include *focus-foci, nucleus-nuclei, alumnus-alumni, fungus-fungi*. Other pluralization processes come from Greek (*criterion-criteria, phenomenon-phenomena*) or Old English (*child-children, ox-oxen*). Because these irregular morphemes deviate from the regular /s/, /z/, /ɪz/ ending of regular plurals, language learners tend to have difficulty with them. You might hear a learner say *childs* for the plural of *child*, for instance. This is not a bad thing; it actually indicates that the learner is picking up on the most frequently used rule for pluralization.

In some cases, entire syntactic processes can change as a result of borrowing. This process takes longer than lexical borrowing, but once it occurs it is the most drastic modifier of a language. For instance, in Romansch, a language spoken in Switzerland, noun phrases were historically structured as noun + adjective, as in *shirt blue* or *shoe small*. However, with extensive contact with

German, over time the entire shape of the noun phrase in Romansch shifted to adjective + noun, as in *blue shirt* and *small shoe*. Changing the shape of the noun phrase structure rule can make quite a striking difference in the language.

The important takeaway in understanding borrowing is that this is a natural process. Although the reasons for language change can vary from innocuous to heinous, the process of language change as a function of language contact is a natural process. Though people might dislike language change, it has been occurring since the very beginning of the history of language. So long as languages meet other languages, they will influence one another. Borrowing is just one facet of that.

8.4 Pidgins

Earlier, we talked about various language contact situations, such as trade, migration, and conquest. Let us consider the first example: trade. Suppose there is a community on one side of a river and another community on the other side. Previously, they had not been in contact due to the dangerous raging river, but prolonged drought caused the river to dry up and people can now easily travel to the other side. When the two communities come into contact, they find that each community speaks a language that is unintelligible to the other. However, they also learn that they each have resources that would be beneficial to the other community, and doing business with one another would serve everyone well. To conduct business, they must communicate, and while at first they could get away with nonlinguistic interactions involving gestures, this rudimentary communication is rather limited and unsustainable. Thus, a **pidgin** is formed.

A pidgin is a speech form that is primarily used as a means of communication among people who do not share a common language. Pidgins are different from languages in that there are no native speakers. It is used only between people who need to communicate past a language barrier, and the speakers of either language would not use it amongst themselves. In the event that there is an unequal balance of power between the groups that come into contact, the language spoken by the people in power is called the **superstrate** language, and the language spoken by the less powerful people is called the **substrate** language. In the pidgin that develops as a result of contact with power imbalances, the superstrate language is typically the one that provides a large percentage of the vocabulary. This is called a **lexifier**, or the language that contributes the most vocabulary. The substrate language typically influences the phonetics and phonology of the pidgin. Thus, a pidgin might be more intelligible to the speakers of the superstrate language, but sound more like the substrate language.

Let us return to the trade scenario. At first, linguistic communication between the two communities might occur by creating a few words that pertain only to their business of trade. This is the **jargon stage** of pidgin formation, where there is a small collection of words that are limited to one specific purpose.

For instance, the pidgin might contain words for numbers (for pricing, counting), names of the resources that are being traded, and a few verbs like *sell* and *buy*, and this jargon might be used among the selected people in each community that interface with the other community. At the jargon stage, there are many inconsistencies from day to day and from person to person. Two people engaged in a trade negotiation might use one set of jargon that works for them, but the next time they meet they might use another set of words. Additionally, if another pair of tradespeople are engaged in a conversation, they might use a set of words that is completely different from the one the first pair of people used. In short, there is no established set of vocabulary.

As the business relationship grows, more communication is needed in order to express more complex meanings. This results in a more established and consistent set of words, phrases, and syntax for communication. This stage of pidgin formation is called the **stabilized pidgin** stage. Stabilized pidgins are more consistent from day to day and from person to person. For example, the same vocabulary and structure that Person A and Person B use when conducting negotiations are also used when Person C and Person D are doing business. It is still generally used only for one purpose (e.g., trade), but it has a regular system that allows speakers of two different languages to understand one another when speaking about that specific purpose. As compared to the source languages, pidgins have reduced inflectional and derivational morphology. This means that, for example, morphemes for tense or pluralization are usually simplified or omitted. Additionally, pidgins tend to have simplified phonological systems as compared to the source language. For example, Fijian fricatives /ß/ and /ð/ become stops /b/ and /d/ in Pidgin Fijian, a pidgin that derived from Fijian and English (Muysken & Smith, 1994).

Some stabilized pidgins develop even further in terms of utility; rather than just being reserved for one purpose—such as trade—some pidgins catch on and become used in other realms of life, like education, religion, food, music, or personal relationships. This stage is called the **expanded pidgin** stage, where the pidgin expands its usage across different domains of life. At this point, there might be a great number of people who speak it. It is important to remember, however, that there is still a key distinction between a pidgin and a language. A pidgin does not have any native speakers, while a language does. However expanded it may be, pidgin is still just a communicative tool rather than a language because it is only used to bridge a gap between speakers of two different languages.

8.5 Creoles

The question you may be asking at this point is, when does that pidgin become a language? The answer: it is when babies learn it as their first language. By the time a pidgin becomes a creole, it has developed enough of its own phonetics, phonology, morphology, syntax, semantics, and pragmatics. The brain registers that it is a complex and developed language instead of a rudimentary communication tool and begins to acquire it. This new language is what we call a **creole**. Though you may have heard the word creole being used to refer to a low-status "improper" form of communication, it is actually a fully fledged language as complex and developed as the most high status languages in our world today. A creole is simply a newly formed language that has arisen out of a contact variety, usually from what used to be a pidgin. This process is called **creolization**. Now, however, the language has native speakers for the first time in its history.

Creoles are unique in that there is often a discernable point in history when contact between two languages took place. The contact almost always means there is one socially powerful group that subjugates a less powerful group, as in conquest, slavery, or war. Part of the reason why creoles are generally seen as less prestigious in society is because of this reason; it is often spoken by peoples who are dominated by another group. Additionally, because creoles arise out of contact between the language of the powerful and less powerful groups—the superstrate and substrate languages—the resulting creole sounds like a different version of the source languages. Creoles, like pidgins, have reduced phonology and inflectional morphology as compared to the source languages, so they are somewhat recognizable but sound different. Because of this, society views the creole as less prestigious than the powerful source language, incorrectly believing that the creole is a contaminated or bastardized version of the "real" language. For instance, there are those who view Jamaican Creole as "poor English", but in reality it is a fully fledged language with a complex system of phonetics, phonology, morphology, syntax, semantics, and pragmatics. The perception is based on misunderstanding about its origin and complexity, not reality.

Let us explore the language complexity of Fa d'Ambu, a creole spoken by people of mixed African, Portuguese, and Spanish descent on Annobón Island, off the coast of Equatorial Guinea. The creole was formed during the 16th century when Portuguese settlers arrived in Annobón and forced African slaves to work the plantations on the island (Post, 1994). The creole is thus a contact language derived from Portuguese and West African languages. Fa d'Ambu is still spoken today on the island and on the mainland as well, and is a source of pride among its speakers (Post, 1994). Fa d'Ambu employs a complex syntactic process called serial verb construction, in which multiple verbs are used in a series to convey a singular meaning as in (1):

(1)	Amu	fo	Pale	bi
	I	leave	Pale	come
		"I come from Pale".		

Another sophisticated feature of Fa d'Ambu is that it employs reduplication (see Chapter 4). Reduplication is a process that changes a word's meaning by repeating or copying all or part of the word. In Fa d'Ambu, verbs, nouns, and adjectives can be reduplicated to intensify a meaning (*kitsyi* "small"; *kitsyikitsyi* "very small"), express that something is iterative (*nda* "to walk"; *ndanda* "to stroll"), or to demonstrate a distributive property (*dosy* "two"; *dodosy* "both") (Post, 1994). Reduplication is seen in many of the world's languages, such as Korean and Turkish, and Fa d'Ambu is no different. The main point is that creoles such as Fa d'Ambu still consist of the same regular, systematic features that socially prominent languages have, and linguistically it is no better or worse, no more or less developed than any other language in the world.

Voices From the Classroom 8.1—Affirming Speakers of Minority Languages

Growing up Hispanic in the U.S. trained me to really value the retention of my Spanish in the context of the influences of English hegemony. Thus, when I taught a high school ESL class with several Guatemalan students, I felt it necessary to encourage them to retain their Spanish too. But my students did not just speak Spanish as their heritage language, they also spoke Q'anjob'al, a Mayan language. It was then that I recognized that although the Spanish language occupies a minority status in the U.S., it too produces hegemonic effects in Latin America and thus contributes to the erasure of indigenous people's language and culture. I realized the importance of recognizing the treatment of minority languages outside of the U.S. because students will likely bring these influences with them into your classroom and it's important to validate all of their languages, not just the colonial ones.

Jazmín Brito, High School ESL Teacher

8.6 World Englishes

English is a global language in today's world. In fact, there are more second language speakers of English than there are native speakers of the language. It is no wonder, then, that there are many varieties of English spoken throughout the world, even in countries that we do not normally think of as English-speaking countries. When students are learning English, they think of it as a uniform, standardized language. However, the truth is, English has had so much contact with so much of the world, and the number of speakers—if you count both native and nonnative—amount to about a fifth of the entire planet. English is anything but uniform because of the vast number of people that speak it and the diverse contact it has had with other languages of the world.

According to Kachru (1985), **World Englishes** are international varieties of English spoken in three circles: the inner circle, the outer circle, and the expanding circle. As can be seen in Figure 8.1, the inner circle consists of countries like the U.S., Canada, U.K., Australia, and New Zealand, where English is typically learned as a first language. The outer circle, which includes places like India, Malaysia, Kenya, Singapore, and the Philippines, describes countries where English is most everybody's second language (**L2**) or second first language (**L1**), and it is used as the **lingua franca**, or common language spoken between different language communities. The expanding circle is even bigger, encompassing countries where English is used for specific purposes. These countries include China, Korea, Russia, Egypt, Indonesia, and Taiwan.

World Englishes make up a large category of creoles, in which English and another language come into contact to form a new and different language. They are fully fledged languages in their own right, and they are not "deviations from the norm". Due to the global nature of World Englishes, each variety takes linguistic features from the local or indigenous languages in the surrounding areas. One such example is Singlish. Singlish is a World English spoken in Singapore, and derives from Malay, Mandarin Chinese, Tamil, and English. Speakers of American English or British English may be able to understand

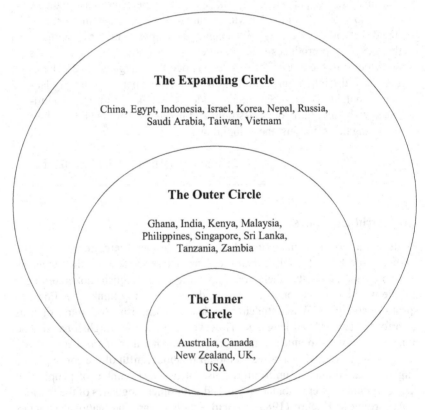

The Expanding Circle

China, Egypt, Indonesia, Israel, Korea, Nepal, Russia,
Saudi Arabia, Taiwan, Vietnam

The Outer Circle

Ghana, India, Kenya, Malaysia,
Philippines, Singapore, Sri Lanka,
Tanzania, Zambia

The Inner
Circle

Australia, Canada
New Zealand, UK,
USA

Figure 8.1 The Three Concentric Circles of English

Source: Adapted from Kachru (1985)

some snippets of Singlish, but would have difficulty with full comprehension because of the influence of the other origins of this unique World English.

For instance, Singlish uses an array of sentence-final particles that convey subtle meaning. Adding *lah* to the end of a sentence can soften the tone and make you sound more apologetic, but it can also turn the utterance into a command. The addition of *hor* to the end of a sentence indicates that the speaker is requesting confirmation or agreement, and adding *meh* denotes incredulity. Singlish also has reduplication for emphasis: e.g., *hot* "hot", *hothot* "very hot". Because Singapore is a diverse country with people of many different backgrounds, the common language of Singlish is a powerful marker of identity and belongingness. Although some people with prescriptive views discount the language as a bastardization of "pure English", the structure of Singlish is quite sophisticated and highly complex.

Notice that there is a difference between L2 English and World English. L2 English speakers are in the process of learning English as a second language and are nonnative speakers of the language. They do not have native-like competence (yet). However, World English speakers are quite different: they grow up speaking English in their home country, so they are very comfortable speaking it and would even consider it their L1. The interesting question to consider is, are students who come from outer and expanding circles English learners? In other words, if they have spoken a World English all their lives, then move to the U.S. and enter school there, should the school place them in an ESL class, or in a mainstream class without any language support?

From one point of view, they are absolutely English speakers, just not speakers of the variety of English that is being used at school. They are also certainly not like students who come to school with no English background whatsoever. They are fully proficient native speakers of their variety of English. However, the other side of the coin is to examine how different the World English is from the English used in American schools. In Chapter 7 we talked about how some nonstandard varieties like African American English, while mutually intelligible with Mainstream American English, have key differences that sometimes go unnoticed by teachers as an area of difficulty. Teachers might incorrectly assume that the students are not performing well because they "speak poorly", but the reason is that they speak another language. It might look and sound like English, but it's another language in many ways.

As we have seen, World Englishes differ in terms of sounds, words, grammar, etc. While World English speakers do not need the kind of ESL curriculum that an L2 English speaker needs, if the World English is significantly different, there may be a need for guidance to transition from one language to another. This is where the linguist-teacher comes in; having the ability to identify differences between two languages and specifically target them (e.g., one is a null copula language, the other is not), the teacher can discern what is needed to help students bridge the gap between the English they speak and the English that is used at school. It also helps that the teacher realizes that it is difference, not deficiency, that characterizes the variety of English the student speaks. World English speakers speak a contact variety of English that has influence from other local or indigenous languages, not a bastardized or erroneous version of the "correct" English. Being aware of these linguistic differences helps teachers better serve students who come from these backgrounds.

Further Reading

Muysken, P., Arends, J., & Smith, N. (Eds.). (1995). *Pidgins and creoles: An introduction.* Amsterdam: John Benjamins.
Velupillai, V. (2015). *Pidgins, creoles and mixed languages: An introduction.* Amsterdam: John Benjamins Publishing Company.

Exercises

1. Choose five words from your native or target language and look up the etymology of the words. What were the origins of the words, and what other languages influenced them? Listed are two examples you can follow.

   Word: cotton
   Etymology: Middle English *coton*, from Anglo-French *cotun*, from Old Italian *cotone*, from Arabic *quṭun, quṭn*

   Word: river
   Etymology: Middle English *rivere*, from Anglo-French, from Vulgar Latin **riparia*, from Latin, feminine of *riparius* riparian, from *ripa* bank, shore; perhaps akin to Greek *ereipein* to tear down

2. Sranan is a creole spoken in Surinam, South America. Sranan is influenced by English, Dutch, West African languages, and Caribbean English-based creoles (Adamson & Smith, 1994).

taki "speak"	taki-maN "speaker"
wroko "work"	wroko-maN "worker"
siki "sick"	siki-maN "sick person"
blaka "black"	blaka-maN "black person"
bere "belly"	bere-maN "pregnant woman"
boto "boat"	boto-maN "boatman"
lobi "love"	lobi-waN "loved one"
ferfi "paint"	ferfi-waN "painted one"
tranga "strong"	tranga-waN "strong one"
siki "sick"	siki-waN "sick one"
baka "back"	baka-waN "(the) one behind"
sey-waN "(the) one at the side"	sey "side"

   (Adamson & Smith, 1994)

Consider the preceding data set and answer the following questions.

a. What is the lexifier language? How do you know?
b. What does the -maN suffix do in Sranan?
c. What does the -waN suffix do in Sranan?
d. Based on the phonological patterns you see in the preceding data set, what is the English translation for the following Sranan words?

  (a) hebi
  (b) fatu
  (c) brada
  (d) dringi
  (e) lafu

3. Choose a word or phrase that is widely known and recognized throughout the world. A good choice might be a celebrity's name, a popular food, or city. Find video clips online of speakers of five different languages saying the word or phrase. Use IPA to transcribe the way it is pronounced in those five languages, and identify the differences. What does it reveal about the phonological rules about each language?

References

Adamson, L., & Smith, N. (1994). Sranan. In J. Arends, P. Muysken, & N. Smith (Eds.), *Pidgins and creoles: An introduction* (pp. 219–232). Amsterdam and Philadelphia: John Benjamins Publishing Company.

Kachru, B. (1985). Standards, codification and sociolinguistic realism: The English language in the outer circle. In R. Quirk & H. G. Widdowson (Eds.), *English in the world: Teaching and learning the language and literatures* (pp. 11–30). Retrieved from www.jstor.org/stable/326771?origin=crossref

Muysken, P., & Smith, N. (1994). The study of pidgin and creole languages. In J. Arends, P. Muysken, & N. Smith (Eds.), *Pidgins and creoles: An introduction* (pp. 3–14). Amsterdam and Philadelphia: John Benjamins Publishing Company.

Post, M. (1994). Fa d'Ambu. In J. Arends, P. Muysken, & N. Smith (Eds.), *Pidgins and creoles: An introduction* (pp. 191–204). Amsterdam and Philadelphia: John Benjamins Publishing Company.

9 History of English

9.1 Introduction

All languages change over time. Because humans are the carriers of language—and humans and their behavior constantly change—so language does too. In Chapter 7 we talked about how languages vary across time and space, and in Chapter 8 we learned about the ways in which languages can change shape due to contact with other languages. Change is simply a natural characteristic of human language; in fact, the only time a language does not change is when all its speakers are deceased. Even languages that have official academies that regulate the vocabulary, grammar, and usage of the language still experience change over time. Of course, humans can influence the way that this change happens—pushing it in one way or the other—but these influences still cannot quell the natural progression of a language.

The English that we speak today is the result of a long history. It is a language that has changed through much contact with various European languages and has seen dynamic changes throughout its past. Contrary to what prescriptivists and other like-minded folks will have you believe, there is no such thing as "pure" English. In fact, if we were to look at the breakdown of the genealogy of English the way you would a dog, English would be considered a good old mutt. English has influence from German, French, Scandinavian languages, Latin, Arabic, Greek, Czech, Hebrew, and a host of other languages. Additionally, English has changed so much in the last few centuries that if we were to listen to a clip of Old English or Middle English, we would not be able to understand it at all.

Most linguists divide English into roughly four historical phases: Prehistory (to c. 450), **Old English** (c. 450–c. 1150), **Middle English** (c. 1150–c. 1450), and **Modern English** (c. 1450–present). This chapter shows the extensive phonological and grammatical changes English has undergone throughout its history, often as a result of contact with other languages such as Old Norse, French, and Latin. It also explains the role of the printing press in stabilizing English spelling.

9.2 Prehistory (to c. 450)

The languages spoken by the original inhabitants of the British Isles belonged to the Celtic (pronounced /kɛltɪk/) family. Modern-day examples of Celtic languages include Gaelic (in Ireland), Welsh (in Wales), and Breton (in Northern France). The Celts had come to the islands around the middle of the first millennium BC and were, in turn, subjugated by the Romans, who arrived in 43 BC. While the Romans were initially reluctant to colonize this land, they did ultimately occupy Britain in a serious way, and introduced Christianity. The main Roman era spanned two centuries, from c. 200 to c. 400. As the Roman Empire came under increasing attack from the Goths and other tribes, however, the Romans retreated closer and closer to home, abandoning their more far-flung colonies. By 410, the Roman armies had left the British Isles to help defend their empire in Europe.

Neglected by the Romans, the British Celts turned to powerful Germanic tribes for protection. The Jutes, the first group to arrive, came from Jutland, in the northern part of modern-day Denmark, and settled in southern and southeastern Britain. Later, the Angles and the Saxons came from the south of the Danish peninsula and settled in Britain. While the Celts looked to these Germanic tribes to fight for them, the real intentions of the new settlers were to enslave the Celtic natives. The Germanic invaders savagely destroyed or pushed back the Celtic communities into areas like Cornwall, Wales, Cumbria, and the Scottish borders. Adding insult to injury, the German invaders even called the native Celts *wealas* ("foreigners"), from which the name Welsh is derived. The result of this turbulent period was that Britain became a predominantly Anglo-Saxon culture. Today, relatively few vestiges of Celtic culture survive.

The Angles, Saxons, and Jutes all spoke a Germanic tongue in different dialects. Because most people during this time lived in small, self-contained villages and traveled only short distances, dialects were numerous, and there were relatively few opportunities for speakers of one dialect to be influenced by speakers of another. However, we do ultimately see the development of a recognizable Old English language by the end of this period.

9.3 Old English (c. 450–c. 1150)

Old English was highly Germanic in vocabulary and syntax, and inflected. What does it mean for a language to be inflected? Whereas Modern English depends primarily on word order to clarify grammatical relations, Old English required different grammatical markers to show whether a given noun was, say, a subject or an object. For example, consider the following two sentences in Old English:

(1)	*Se*	*cyning*	*meteth*	*thone*	*biscop.*
	the	king	meets	the	bishop

("The king meets the bishop".)

(2)	*Thone*	*biscop*	*meteth*	*se*	*cyning.*
	the	bishop	meets	the	king

("The king meets the bishop".)

Notice that both (1) and (2) mean "The king meets the bishop". How is this possible? The answer lies in grammatical inflection. **Inflection** is a process of word formation, in which a word is modified to express different grammatical categories such as tense, case, voice, aspect, number, and gender. In (1) and (2), we know that the king is the subject of both sentences because it is preceded by a subject marker *se*. Similarly, we know that the bishop is the object of both (1) and (2) because it is preceded by an object marker *thone*. The reason Old English order could vary as in (1) and (2) is that the relationships between the different parts of the sentence were signaled by these inflections. Over time, however, inflection was lost, and word order became much more important (see 9.4 Middle English).

The history of Old English vocabulary is characterized by repeated invasions, with newcomers to the islands bringing their own languages with them and infusing their vocabulary into English. There were two major lexical invasions during this period—one from Latin and the other from Norse. Latin vocabulary was introduced mainly by Christian missionaries from Ireland and Rome, who brought with them words having to do with the Church, theology, and learning. Words like *altar, apostle, cross, paradise*, and *sabbath* were all borrowed into English from Latin. In addition to religious vocabulary, there were many words having to do with biology that came from Latin during this time such as *plant, organ, rose*, and *dolphin*.

The second major linguistic invasion came as a result of the Viking raids on the British Isles, which began in 787 and continued for some 200 years. As the Danes began to settle down, many places with Danish names appeared in eastern England. Place names that end in -*by* (the Old Norse word for "farm" or "town"), as in *Derby, Whitby*, and *Kerby*, as well as those that end in -*thorpe* ("village"), as in *Scunthorpe, Kettlethorpe*, and *Austhorp*, appeared. The Anglo-Saxons and the Danish settlers had close contact, leading to extensive borrowings. Some of the most common Modern English words were borrowed from Norse at this time, such as *want, take, trust, again*, and *get*. Norse also had a profound effect on the personal pronouns that English uses today (*they, them*, and *their* are all of Norse-origin and replaced the Old English *hī, hēō*, and *hira*). The verb *to be* is also of Norse-origin and replaced the earlier Old English forms.

The period we call Old English spans seven centuries, from c. 450 to c. 1150. Toward the end of this period, Britain was invaded yet again, this time by the Normans who came from modern-day France. The initial linguistic effect of the Norman invasion of 1066 was not that substantial. The Normans mostly kept to themselves as a ruling class, mixing little with their Anglo-Saxon subjects, who in turn had no incentive to learn the language of their rulers. In addition, few members of either group could read. This division between the rulers and the ruled remains very clear to this day, owing to the difference between Anglo-Saxon and Norman-French vocabulary groups in Modern English. For instance, we can think of such terms for animals as *swine, cow, calf, sheep, and deer*—all Anglo-Saxon names, reflecting the fact that the work of livestock-tending was done mostly by the Anglo-Saxons subjects. And we can think of such food terms as *pork, beef, veal, mutton, and venison*—all Norman-French names, reflecting the fact that the Norman invaders led the high life. To the extent that there was any contact between these two groups at this early stage, those Old English speakers who wished to give themselves airs sprinkled their speech with French, as many English speakers do today.

9.4 Middle English (c. 1150–c. 1450)

The Norman invasion was a major event in the history of English. Without the Norman invasion, English would have retained most grammatical inflections and a predominantly Germanic vocabulary. English would have lacked the greatest part of French words that make it seem more like a Romance language today than a Germanic language. It has been estimated that some 10,000 French words came into English during the 13th century. The fact that English is a particularly synonym-rich language, with a vocabulary size twice that of French or Italian or German, owes itself to this massive borrowing. But how was this possible, given the initially minimal contact between the Anglo-Saxons and the Normans? The answer is that when Normandy itself was invaded and taken over, the British Normans found themselves cut off from their home culture, and began assimilating to a greater degree. At the same time, burgeoning commerce was increasingly breaking down barriers between villages and bringing people together.

Britain had three languages that were used in different social domains during this time. French had the world of the court as its chief domain, whereas Latin was used in the Church and legal matters, and Old English was used in everyday speech. But French vocabulary and syntax had begun to exert an increasingly profound influence in these and other domains, and we see this as a defining characteristic of Middle English. French influence on English vocabulary can be seen in the following examples:

a. government—state, empire, statute, treasurer, governor, parliament
b. religion—theology, sermon, baptism, faith, temptation, immortality
c. law—bar, plea, suit, judge, jury, arrest, accuse, crime, trespass
d. colors—blue, vermilion, scarlet, rose
e. food—appetite, cream, dinner, fruit, gravy, salad, sugar, toast
f. home—chair, chamber, lamp, tower, pillar, chimney, cellar
g. the arts—art, beauty, dance, image, literature, music, poet, prose
h. the sciences—anatomy, medicine, plague, poison, stomach, sulphur
i. verbs—change, continue, advise, inform, marry, obey, move, pass, reply
j. adjectives—common, clear, gentle, natural, original, perfect, simple, usual
k. nouns—affection, age, courage, error, hour, mountain, people, river, season

In addition, Old English/French word pairs such as old/ancient, beseech/ pray, house/mansion, and heal/cure show how English words and their French equivalents came to coexist with slightly different connotations.

We can also see traces of both French and Anglo-Saxon influences in plural formations. The -*s* ending of such words as *boy-s* and *girl-s* is characteristic of French while the -*en* ending of such words as *brether-en* and *ox-en* is typical of Anglo-Saxon. But the most important grammatical development during the Middle English period was the establishment of a fixed word order. There was already a tendency toward Subject-Verb-Object (SVO) order in Old English, but this became more firmly established during the Middle English period. As mentioned earlier, Old English used inflections to signal grammatical relationships of words in a sentence. For example, the Old English noun *cyning* ("king") could have different noun endings (-*es*, -*a*, -*e*, and -*um*), as in *cyninges* ("of the king"), *cyninga* ("of the kings"), *cyninge* ("to the king"), or *cyningum* ("to the kings"). But as these word endings gradually disappeared, prepositions became much more important.

9.5 Modern English (c. 1450–Present)

Most linguists divide the Modern English period into Early Modern (c. 1450 to c. 1800) and Modern (c. 1800 to present). In the Early Modern period, English continues to change in significant ways, and there are many points of difference with modern usage. But by the end of the 18th century, the spelling, punctuation, and grammar are very close to what we have in English today. For instance, most people find reading a novel by Jane Austen (1775–1817) relatively straightforward. We can read for pages before encountering somewhat unfamiliar vocabulary and idiomatic expressions. But the same cannot be said about the works by William Shakespeare (1564–1616), which most certainly require us to consult a special edition or a commentary in order to understand the text.

The Early Modern English period begins with the advent of printing in 1476. The invention of the printing press played a key role in the formation of a standard language, which we will discuss in further detail in Section 9.6. For now, the important takeaway is that as a result of the printing press, during the 16th century, there was a flood of new publications in English, prompted by an increasing interest in the classical languages and literatures, science, medicine, and the arts. The period covering two centuries from the invention of the printing press is also called the "Renaissance", and it included the Reformation, the Copernican revolution, and the European colonization of Africa and the Americas.

How did English develop during the Renaissance? Since there weren't adequate words in the language to talk accurately about the new concepts and inventions that were coming out, writers began to borrow them from other languages. Most of the words that entered English at this time were taken from Latin, Greek, French, Italian, Spanish, and Portuguese. And as the age of European colonialism got under way, words came into English from over 50 languages spoken in North America, Africa, and Asia. Some words came directly into English while others came indirectly from Latin or Italian or French. Pronouns underwent significant change, too. While *ye* was used as a subject and *you* as an object in Middle English, *you* became the single form for both subject and object in Early Modern English.

In terms of grammar, constructions involving a double negative (*I cannot do no more*) or impersonal verbs (*me thinks she did*) were common in English during the Renaissance. But beginning in the 1700s, language purists proclaimed that the double negative, or negative concord, was illogical and improper in English (see Chapter 7 for more on negative concord). There were other major efforts to impose order on the language. For one, the completion of *A Dictionary of the English Language* by Samuel Johnson in 1755 had a stabilizing effect on how words were spelled. In addition, many spelling guides were published during the 17th century, which regularized orthography. While variant spellings tended to be socially tolerated during the Renaissance, more strict notions of correctness emerged by the end of the Early Modern English period, and poor spelling became stigmatized.

9.6 The Great Vowel Shift

One of the most profound changes in the history of English is the **Great Vowel Shift**, which occurred during the 14th through 17th century. The Great Vowel Shift was a massive sound change that marks the transition from Middle English to Early Modern English. Essentially, the vowels that had previously been pronounced in one part of the mouth shifted to a different—usually higher—part of the mouth. Before the Great Vowel Shift took place, English consisted of long vowels /i/, /e/, /a/, /o/, /u/. During the Great Vowel Shift, the following eight changes occurred:

Change 1: /i/ and /u/ became diphthongs /əi/ and /əu/, respectively
Change 2: Mid vowels /e/ and /o/ became /i/ and /u/, respectively
Change 3: Low back vowel /a/ became a low front vowel /æ/
Change 4: Mid lax vowels /ɛ/ and /ɔ/ became /e/ and /o/, respectively
Change 5: Low front vowel /æ/ moved up to /ɛ/
Change 6: /e/ moved up to /i/
Change 7: /ɛ/ moved up to /e/
Change 8: /əi/ and /əu/ became /ai/ and /au/, respectively

Figure 9.1 illustrates the changes that occurred in the Great Vowel Shift using the vowel chart.

Some examples from before and after the Great Vowel Shift can be seen in Table 9.1.

Although this historical phenomenon may seem like just some vowels moving around in the mouth, the Great Vowel Shift made English what it is today. There are three main reasons the Great Vowel Shift is deemed to be such a "great" phenomenon. One reason is the speed at which the Great Vowel Shift happened. The fact that this vowel shift occurred across about 400 years is quite unusual and relatively fast as far as language shifts go. Another notable

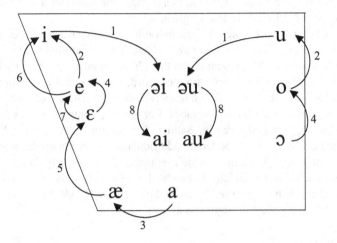

Figure 9.1 The Great Vowel Shift

characteristic is that the Great Vowel Shift did not just affect one vowel—a common occurrence for all languages—but rather it affected nearly *all* the vowels around the same time. Because every word in the English language contains a vowel sound, this means the Great Vowel Shift affected nearly every word in the English language. This was a profound transformation and a reason why Middle English is not mutually intelligible with Modern English. Finally, the Great Vowel Shift is particularly notable because some vowels went through more than one change during this relatively short span of time. For instance, the first example in Table 9.1 shows that the word *bite* was pronounced as /bitə/ in Middle English. During the Great Vowel Shift, the /i/ sound became /əi/ at first, so that /bitə/ became /bəit/ (the final /ə/ was dropped). This is described in Change 1. However, that newly minted /əi/ shifted again to /ai/, such that /bəit/ became /bait/, which is how we pronounce *bite* today. This multistage sound change adds to the complexity and significance of the Great Vowel Shift in the history of the English language.

What could cause such a profound shift in the language? While the exact cause is not known, some scholars have argued that the rapid migration of

Table 9.1 The Great Vowel Shift: Example Words

Gloss	Before the Great Vowel Shift	After the Great Vowel Shift
"bite"	/bitə/	/bait/
"beat"	/bɛtə/	/bit/
"meat"	/mɛt/	/mit/
"moon"	/mon/	/mun/
"house"	/hus/	/haus/

peoples from northern England to the southeast following the Black Death caused a mixing of accents that forced a change in the standard London vernacular. Others have argued that massive borrowing from French was a major factor in the shift. As we discussed in Chapter 8, the meeting of different languages and dialects usually causes language change, and scholars theorize that this might have been the catalyst for the Great Vowel Shift.

What does this have to do with teaching English? Many people are aware that there are significant inconsistencies between spoken English pronunciation and written English spelling. The same *oo* in fl<u>oo</u>d, g<u>oo</u>d, and m<u>oo</u>se is pronounced three different ways: /ʌ/, /ʊ/, and /u/ as in /flʌd/, /gʊd/, and /mus/. These kinds of inconsistencies between pronunciation and spelling make learning to read and write English challenging for even native speakers, and why spelling rules have so many exceptions. If you look up "English spelling" online, many of the search hits will deem the spelling system as broken, absurd, or insane. However, there is a reason behind the seemingly chaotic English spelling system, and this reason is directly linked to the Great Vowel Shift. In the 1400s, just as the Great Vowel Shift was starting to take its course, the printing press was invented, as we discussed earlier. Prior to this point in history, there was less consistency in English spelling because people spelled words the way they were pronounced. Thus, depending on the dialect of English you spoke, words were spelled differently. Once the printing press was invented, however, there was a need to make the spelling more consistent. Unfortunately, this stabilization happened just before English underwent the massive pronunciation shift we just talked about. For example, the printing press used double letters for the long vowels that are so characteristic of Middle English: words like *food* /fod/ was spelled with two *o*'s to represent the long vowel. However, with the Great Vowel Shift, the pronunciation of *food* /fod/ became /fud/, while the spelling, immortalized by the stabilizing printing press, remained *food*.

Although the invention of the printing press is partially responsible for this mismatch between written and spoken English, it also led to the rise of English literacy, an important characteristic of the Renaissance period. Since printed material could be more easily circulated and was easier to reproduce than handwritten documents, more people had access to writing. Literacy was no longer only reserved for religious purposes; writing was used for commerce, literature, and diplomacy. Perhaps more importantly, writing was accessible to everyone, not just the elite. It became more commonplace for middle class children to learn to read and write in school. Having the ability to print books and distribute them led to a wider base of readers and writers than English had ever known before. Thus, the advent of the printing press had significant impact on the culture and tradition of literacy in the English language.

9.7 Northern Cities Chain Shift

A more contemporary example of language change in English is the **Northern Cities Chain Shift**. **Chain shifts** are changes in historical phonology in which one sound influences the change of another, forming a chain reaction. Like with the Great Vowel Shift example, vowels tend to undergo more changes because they are formed and differentiated by tiny changes in the tongue position. Consequently, these vowel changes make a bigger impact because the smallest change in tongue position can completely change the pronunciation of a word. The Northern Cities Chain Shift is a currently ongoing process that is affecting six vowels in the upper Midwest region of the United States, in cities along the Great Lakes. The cities whose speakers are affected by the shift include Buffalo, Detroit, Chicago, Cleveland, Milwaukee, Rochester, and Syracuse. The Northern Cities Chain Shift consists of the following six changes:

Change 1: /æ/ is raised to /eə/ or /ɪə/
Change 2: /ɑ/ is fronted to /æ/
Change 3: /ɔ/ is lowered to /ɑ/
Change 4: /ɛ/ is backed to /ʌ/
Change 5: /ʌ/ is backed to /ɔ/
Change 6: /ɪ/ is lowered to /ɛ/

These six changes can be seen on the vowel chart in Figure 9.2. Examples can be found in Table 9.2.

For example, a speaker who is affected by the Northern Cities Chain Shift may pronounce *bat* as more like *byat* or *hit* as more like *het*. Often, this dialect is characterized by non-Midwesterners as sounding "nasal"; technically, the vowels only sound that way to outsiders because of the raised and fronted changes (Changes 1 and 2). Change 3 is sometimes referred to as the *cot-caught* merger, where the words *cot* and *caught* or *bot* and *bought* are pronounced identically for some speakers.

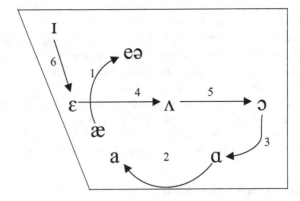

Figure 9.2 Northern Cities Chain Shift Vowel Chart

Table 9.2 Northern Cities Chain Shift: Example Words

Change	Gloss	Other American English	Northern Cities Chain Shift
1	"bat"	[bæt]	[beət] or [bɪət]
2	"lot"	[lɑt]	[læt]
3	"bought"	[bɔt]	[bɑt]
4	"set"	[set] or [sɛt]	[sʌt]
5	"but"	[bʌt]	[bɔt]
6	"hit"	[hɪt]	[hɛt]

It is important to keep in mind that unlike the Great Vowel Shift, which happened centuries ago, the changes in the Northern Cities Chain Shift are currently ongoing. This means that linguists are not certain whether the vowels affected by the Northern Cities Chain Shift will remain where they are or whether they will continue to change. If you encounter a speaker influenced by this chain shift, you might hear that the change is not as extreme as the examples in the rightmost column of Table 9.2, but that it is somewhere on the spectrum. It is also important to remember that the change is not uniform; not all speakers will exhibit all six changes. The Northern Cities Chain Shift, rather, is an overall description of the tendency that linguists are seeing across the region.

For language learners and teachers, this may seem initially problematic. How does one learn and teach English if it is constantly changing? This is another reason why it is helpful for language teachers to be linguists. Linguists know that with language, it is not always a strict dichotomy between correct and incorrect. It is not like math where two plus two really only has one answer. Rather, language comprises a spectrum of variation: pronouncing *bat* as [beət] will work, as will [bæt] and [bat]. Our role as language teachers is to guide learners toward what is typically acceptable for the current time period—it would not be particularly useful for ESL students to learn conversational Middle English, though it would be fun—and also what is typically acceptable for the language environment they are in. It actually does students a disservice if we only expose them to one variety and establish the illusion that English is uniform, unchanging, and rigid. As it has done and will always do, English will continue to change. No language academy, dictionary, or printing press can stop its natural progression.

Recommended Websites

Listen to Beowulf being read in Old English
www.telegraph.co.uk/culture/culturevideo/booksvideo/8135302/Beowulf-reading-in-Old-English-with-translation.html

Exercises

1. Following are several words from Middle English, the way they were pronounced prior to the Great Vowel Shift. Use the vowel chart in Figure 9.1 to determine the sound change(s) that occurred for each word during the Great Vowel Shift. Write the word in Modern English and the sound change(s) the vowels underwent. Hint: word final /ə/ was often dropped.

 a. [tid]
 b. [namə]
 c. [bot]
 d. [abutə]
 e. [bet]

2. Following is the Lord's Prayer in Modern English, Middle English, and Old English. In the table that follows, write the words that you can recognize in each version in the appropriate column. Look at the similarities and differences in the spellings and try to sound out the words in Middle and Old English to see how the language has evolved.

 a. Modern English

 Our Father, who art in heaven, Hallowed be thy Name. Thy kingdom come; thy will be done, on earth as it is in heaven. Give us this day our daily bread, and forgive us our trespasses, as we forgive those who trespass against us, and lead us not into temptation, but deliver us from evil. Amen.

 b. Middle English

 Oure fadir that art in heuenes, halewid be thi name; thi kyngdoom come to; be thi wille don, in erthe as in heuene. Yyue to vs this dai oure breed ouer othir substaunce, and foryyue to vs oure dettis, as we foryyuen to oure dettouris; and lede vs not in to temptacioun, but delyuere vs fro yuel. Amen.

 c. Old English

 Fæder ure þu þe eart on heofonum, Si þin nama gehalgod; to becume þin rice; gewurþe ðin willa, on eorðan swa on heofonum. Urne gedæghwamlican hlaf syle us todæg, and forgyf us ure gyltas swa we forgyfað urum gyltendum; and ne gelæd þu us on costnunge, ac alys us of yfele. Soþlice

 Note: Thorn <þ> and eth <ð> were alternative spellings for the sounds [θ] or [ð]. The symbol <æ> represented a pronunciation in Old English much like the vowel in *cat*.

Modern English	Middle English	Old English
father	fadir	fæder
heaven	heuenes	heofonum

3. All the following listed words have been borrowed into English from other languages. Make an educated guess as to the likely source language for each word. Then look up the etymology of each word in the dictionary to see if your guess was correct.

   a. entrepreneur
   b. renaissance
   c. macho
   d. plaza
   e. cigar
   f. guru
   g. mosquito
   h. lemon
   i. alma mater
   j. typhoon
   k. democracy

4. Following are several examples of English words in the Northern Cities dialect. Use the vowel chart in Figure 9.2 to determine the sound change(s) that occurred for each word during the Northern Cities Chain Shift. Write the word and the sound change(s) the vowels underwent.

   a. [beəg]
   b. [pæt]
   c. [lʌt]
   d. [bɛg]
   e. [pɑ]

10 Bilingualism and Language Policy

10.1 Introduction

The ability to use two or more languages is a valuable asset in today's world. Since social interactions and information exchange increasingly take place across national and linguistic borders, people who possess bilingual competence have a clear advantage over those who don't. Knowing another language opens doors to new worlds and connects you with people from different places. Bilinguals have been shown to demonstrate greater cognitive flexibility and cross-cultural competence than monolinguals. Being bilingual has economic advantages, too, with more job opportunities and better earning potential. It is no wonder then that so many parents are interested in raising bilingual children. Some parents hire bilingual babysitters, others enroll their children in a language immersion program, or play foreign language videos in the hope that an early exposure to another language will help their children learn it.

But what does it mean for people to learn and live with two or more languages? Despite the well-intentioned efforts of many parents, not all children who are exposed to two languages become bilingual. Why do some children become bilingual and others don't? What does it take to raise children bilingually in monolingual societies? In this chapter, we will explore various descriptions of bilingualism and clarify some common misconceptions. We will address questions such as: who is a bilingual? What criteria should be used to define a bilingual? Does one need to have equal proficiency in both languages to be considered a bilingual? Are there different degrees of bilingualism that can vary over time and with circumstances?

We will first look at how prevalent bilingualism (and for that matter, multilingualism) is in the world. Contrary to popular assumptions, bilingualism is not a rare phenomenon. Well more than half the world's population speak two or more languages on a daily basis, and you are in fact in the majority if you speak more than one language.

Many people, when asked about bilingual people, think of simultaneous interpreters who work for the United Nations. UN interpreters are expected to have perfect command of multiple languages and be able to understand and have expressions in another language for any number of issues in a split second. They are expected to interpret a wide range of subjects including politics, legal affairs, economic and social issues, finance, administration, as well as anything else a delegate might say. It takes many years of language study and training to operate at this advanced level. However, these language professionals constitute a tiny minority of the world's bilinguals. The vast majority of the bilinguals in the world do not have perfect command of two languages. In this chapter, we will see why that is the case, and how bilinguals use their two languages, separately or together, for different purposes with different people to accomplish their communicative goals.

We will also explore program options for educating students in more than one language. Besides learning another language through informal interaction in the family and community, children can significantly expand their bilingual capacities by being schooled in two languages. To most people, bilingual education simply means teaching students in two languages. In reality, there is a wide range of program options with various goals, target students, and amount of time spent in instruction in each language.

We will see that different populations require different bilingual approaches. While students who come from majority-language backgrounds tend to learn a second language with no negative consequence to their mother tongue, many minority-language speakers lose their first language in the process of learning the societal language. Schools tend to privilege the views of the dominant groups at the expense of minority groups, and minority-language speakers quickly realize that their languages are not valued in school and the mainstream society. Thus, a successful bilingual education program will often go out of its way to provide extra support for students' development of the societally weaker language. Clearly, educational and policy decisions influence bilingual outcomes, and we will see what teachers, parents, and policy makers can do to promote bilingualism for all kinds of students.

10.2 Prevalence of Bilingualism in the World

The use of two or more languages is an ordinary fact of life for an estimated two thirds of the world's population. There are more than 6,000 languages spoken in the world today and only about 190 countries, which suggests the presence of intense language contact within national borders. No matter where you go in the world, you are likely to find distinct linguistic groups within national borders. In fact, societal use of multiple languages is common in many multilingual countries in Africa, Asia, Europe, and elsewhere. For example, some 79 different languages are spoken in Ghana and 37 in Senegal. In India, 216 languages are spoken by at least 10,000 speakers each, and 24 of these languages are recognized by the national constitution.

Even within the world's so-called monolingual countries, there are substantial numbers of multilingual individuals and communities. For instance, more than 60 million people in the United States—or one in five Americans—aged five or older speak a language other than English at home. Collectively, they speak more than 350 different languages in addition to English (U.S. Census Bureau, 2015). In Germany, more than 16 million people, or over 20% of the total population, have an immigrant background. Many of these individuals are bilingual in German and in their home languages as well.

Although there are more bilingual people in the world than monolinguals, scholars have frequently treated bilingualism as a special case or a deviation from the supposed monolingual norm. Historically, linguistic research has tended to focus on monolinguals and has treated bilinguals and multilinguals as exceptions. For instance, Chomsky's (1965) influential theory of grammar was concerned primarily with "an ideal speaker-listener, in a completely homogeneous speech community, who knows its language perfectly" (p. 3). Given the emphasis on describing the linguistic competence of the ideal monolingual speaker, bilingualism was often treated as a problematic or exceptional form of communication taken up by people who do not seem to know either language fully. This monolingual bias is also evident in popular misconceptions about bilinguals. Let's take a look at a few of them.

10.3 Misconceptions About Bilingualism

One of the most common misconceptions about bilingualism is that a "real" bilingual is completely fluent and equally competent in two languages. Many people think that in order to be considered bilingual, they must have perfect command of two languages like a UN interpreter. In reality, however, bilinguals will rarely have perfectly balanced proficiency in their two languages. Terms such as "full" bilingual and "balanced" bilingual represent idealized concepts that do not characterize most of the world's bilinguals. Put another way, a bilingual is not two monolinguals put together in one person.

Bilingual proficiency is very much a result of experience with the languages in question. Because most people use their two languages for different purposes with different people, bilinguals are rarely completely fluent in two languages. For example, a Chinese-immigrant student in an American school might speak mostly Cantonese at home with her family but use English at school. An Indian businessman living in Mumbai might speak Gujarati, his native language, at home with his family, but use Marathi in the market. With people who don't speak either Gujarati or Marathi, he may speak Hindi, a common language used by speakers of different mother tongues in India. What's important to understand is that the Chinese-immigrant student and the Indian businessman will develop proficiency in each of their languages only to the extent required by their need to communicate in those languages. UN-interpreter-level competence is not required for them to satisfy their communicative needs at home, work, or school.

Another common misconception about bilingualism is that it delays children's language development and puts them at risk of academic failure. Before the 1960s, many studies highlighted the negative effects of bilingualism on children. Observers noted various limitations associated with the language development of bilingual children, such as restricted vocabularies, limited grammatical structures, unusual word order, errors in morphology, hesitations, stuttering, and so on. Some even argued that bilingualism hurt child intelligence and led to split personalities.

In educational circles, some people used the term "semilingual" to describe bilingual students who appear to lack proficiency in both of their languages. A 1996 *Los Angeles Times* article reported that there were 6,800 immigrant-background students in the schools of the Los Angeles Unified School District who were labeled "non-nons" or "clinically disfluent"—that is, children who allegedly did not know English, Spanish, or any other language (cited in Valadez, MacSwan, & Martínez, 2000). In response, Valadez et al. (2000) systematically compared the oral language proficiencies of children who were labeled as "clinical disfluent" by school psychologists and children who were identified as having "normal" or "high" ability.

Valadez et al. (2000) found that the children labeled "clinically disfluent" or "semilingual" did not have a poorer knowledge of morphology and syntax. Contrary to the school evaluations, these students were not inexpressive. In fact, the researchers found that the "semilingual" children had the same command of language as their peers in the control group. Valadez et al. (2000) concluded that labels such as "semilingual" and "non-non" are not based on measured language competencies but rather reflect mainstream society's lack of knowledge about children who come from minority-language-speaking homes. They argue that these terms reflect a widespread monolingual bias in education.

Research comparing monolingual and bilingual children on a wide variety of linguistic and cognitive tasks frequently includes a measure of receptive vocabulary, often the Peabody Picture Vocabulary Test (PPVT). Although many studies have reported lower vocabulary scores for bilingual children than for monolinguals, it is difficult to determine whether the vocabulary difference is due to sampling error because each study is based on a small sample of participants.

To address this problem, Bialystok, Luk, Peets, and Yang (2010) analyzed the PPVT scores of 1,738 Canadian children between three and ten years of age recruited from multiple studies. They found that there was a significant difference in the vocabulary sizes of monolingual and bilingual children. However, the difference was largely limited to words that are part of home life (e.g., *squash, camcorder, pitcher*). This is understandable since English is not used as extensively in bilingual homes as it is in the homes of monolingual English-speaking children. In contrast, when the researchers examined the school vocabulary—words that children would encounter in school (e.g., *astronaut, rectangle, writing*)—the scores for monolingual and bilingual children were more similar. The researchers concluded that bilingual children are thus not disadvantaged in academic and literacy achievement in school.

Some studies found that young immigrant children momentarily lag in grammatical development in both of their languages when compared to their same-age monolingual peers. These differences in grammatical accuracy generally disappear as they grow up. However, findings like these have been misinterpreted as suggesting that bilingualism harms a child's well-being. Similarly, tests that are designed for monolinguals are often used to compare bilinguals' proficiency in either of their languages with that of monolinguals. These assessments do not consider the fact that bilinguals use their two languages with different people, in different contexts, and for different purposes. Again, a bilingual is not the sum of two monolinguals. Thus, it is not accurate to simply add the results from two monolingual tests to measure bilinguals' language ability.

Overall, past research tended to look at bilinguals from a deficit perspective. They looked for what bilinguals cannot do relative to monolinguals. In contrast, much of the current (and more carefully designed) research shows the advantages of bilingualism, for instance, the benefits of bilingualism on children's cognitive development (e.g., Barac, Bialystok, Castro, & Sanchez, 2014). While this bilingual advantage has not been found in all work, the bulk of the existing research has pointed to specific advantages that bilingualism brings.

In many countries, immigrant and minority-language-speaking parents are frequently advised by teachers, doctors, and speech therapists to stop speaking their native languages at home so as not to confuse children with input from two languages. The advice is based on the idea that a mismatch between home language and school language will result in academic difficulties. But the argument that bilingual input confuses children is nonsense since most children growing up in bilingual or multilingual societies (e.g., India, Singapore, and many Asian and African countries) learn to use two or more languages with no negative consequences to their cognitive development. The view that bilingual input confuses children is not supported by empirical linguistic evidence.

Related to this idea is the erroneous view that bilingual speech is a sign of some sort of communicative deficit. **Code-switching** is the alternating use of two or more languages within the same conversation, usually when bilinguals are in the company of other bilinguals. Code-switching is one of the most obvious signs of an individual's bilingual abilities, since very few bilinguals keep their two languages totally separate. However, monolinguals who hear bilinguals code-switch may have negative attitudes toward code-switching and think it indicates lack of mastery of either language. We can see negative attitudes toward bilingual speech in pejorative names people use to refer to the mixed speech of bilinguals, such as Chinglish (Chinese-English), Konglish (Korean-English), and Franglais (French-English). Bilinguals themselves may feel embarrassed about their language mixing behavior and attribute it to carelessness or laziness. However, a large body of research in the past few decades has shown that code-switching, far from being a communicative deficit, is a valuable linguistic strategy.

For example, we now know that code-switching requires unusually high grammatical sensitivity and that individuals who code-switch do not lack syntactic knowledge. Code-switching is not a haphazard mish-mash of two languages, but is rather orderly. Having access to two languages, bilinguals have more ways to convey their meanings than do monolinguals. Bilinguals code-switch to communicate a variety of social meanings, including toning down a statement that might otherwise sound too strong, interjecting to grab the floor in the conversation, and expressing solidarity with members of the same ethnic group. Code-switching may also signal playfulness in some contexts while it can represent a discourse of resistance in others. Bilingual musicians and songwriters use code-switching to push artistic boundaries and reinforce their messages. For instance, in Korean popular music (K-pop), English is mixed to assert "a new identity", enabling Korean youth "to challenge dominant representations of authority, to resist mainstream norms and values, and to reject older generation's conservatism" (Lee, 2004, p. 429).

While research clearly shows that bilinguals' ability to switch between languages is a useful tool, code-switching is generally discouraged by teachers, who often believe that it is distracting and robs students of opportunities to practice the target language. In some ESL classrooms, teachers have a "Speak-Only-English" rule to prevent students from using their home languages. But forcing students to speak only the target language in the classroom is counterproductive because it can prevent students from making connections to what they already know. More importantly, insisting on strictly separating two languages ignores what it means for bilinguals to live with two languages. A bilingual's two languages are not two separate compartments in the brain but are much more interconnected.

10.4 Bilingual Education Programs

Given these facts about bilingualism, what program options are available for attaining bilingualism? As we mentioned earlier, to most people, bilingual education simply means teaching students in two languages. In reality, there is a wide range of program options with various goals, target students, and amount of time spent in instruction in each language. Programs also differ widely in terms of teaching methodologies and how the two languages are perceived by the wider community.

What often makes conversations about bilingual education confusing is that the same terms are used to describe programs with very different goals and outcomes. For example, the term "immersion" can have very different outcomes for different populations. People who have lived in other countries often attest to the usefulness of being immersed in another language. For example, an American college student who spends a year abroad in Mexico, living with a Mexican family and speaking Spanish all the time, might later credit her fluency in Spanish to her language immersion experience. She will have added skills in another language to her existing linguistic repertoire. This is an example of **additive bilingualism**, a situation in which one learns a second language while continuing to use the first language.

In contrast, a young child of Mexican immigrants to the U.S. may experience immersion in English in a quite different way. She is, by definition, a speaker of a minority language. Her home language, Spanish, is not typically valued in school and is looked down on. She feels the pressure to speak only English in the school cafeteria and the playground. Spanish has no place in the school curriculum and she receives little or no support to develop further in it. As she goes through schooling receiving English-only instruction, the effective outcome is not Spanish-English bilingualism, but monolingualism in English. This is an example of **subtractive bilingualism**, a situation in which the socially dominant language replaces the weaker minority language. Immersion in this case leads to a very different outcome than the study abroad example.

In classifying bilingual education programs, it is useful to refer to Cummins's (1996) distinction between the *means* and the *goals* of a particular program. When defined in terms of the means, bilingual education simply refers to the use of two languages in instructional settings. Proficiency in two languages is not necessarily a desired outcome. For example, **transitional bilingual education** programs in the U.S. provide native language instruction to immigrant students only as a temporary bridge to learning English (usually for about one to three years). Once students are deemed to have enough English, the native language is dropped from the curriculum and no further support is provided in the native language. Transitional bilingual education is an example of a **weak form of bilingual education** and often results in subtractive bilingualism.

When defined in terms of goals, however, bilingual education may actually involve teaching students in one language only for some time. For instance, immigrant students may learn their school subjects (e.g., math, science, social studies) almost exclusively in their native language so that they can learn to read and write in the language they already speak. This helps students establish a strong foundation in the minority language, which is weaker and lower in status than the majority language. After the initial grades, as the majority language is gradually added to the curriculum, these programs still maintain close to 50% of instruction in the minority language throughout elementary school. These programs promote additive bilingualism. **Developmental bilingual education** in the U.S. is an example of such a **strong form of bilingual education**.

In 1953, UNESCO published a report titled *The Use of Vernacular Languages in Education*. The UNESCO report stresses the importance of educating students through a language that they understand. For students who come from minority-language backgrounds, this means educating them in their mother tongues. More than sixty years since the publication of this report, there is now a large body of research that shows that teaching students through their native languages helps them develop content knowledge, skills, and literacy, and promotes their learning of additional languages. We also know that developing and maintaining two or more languages over time is associated with multiple health and cognitive advantages, positive emotional and social development, and stronger families and communities. Research clearly points to the benefits of multilingualism for the individual, the family, and the broader society.

Research in educational settings all over the world has shown the benefits of multilingual education programming for all kinds of students, including language-minority and language-majority students as well as Indigenous and refugee students. Research suggests positive outcomes from providing instruction to Indigenous students in their mother tongues, even when it is logistically and financially difficult to do so. For instance, Papua New Guinea is home to about 820 languages spoken by about 4.5 million people. After years of English-only education policy and low youth engagement rates in formal schooling, the government mandated in 1991 that 380 national languages be used as media of instruction for the first three years of formal schooling. Enacted in 1995, the policy provides three years of mother-tongue education as well as instruction in English as a second language. Analysis of the implementation of this policy revealed a number of positive outcomes, including increased access to education, higher literacy rates, and lower dropout rates, particularly among girls (Klaus, 2003).

Bilingual education also has been shown to be beneficial for Indigenous children in the U.S. who may no longer speak their Native language (e.g., Dakota, Navajo, or Ojibwe) at home. Indigenous children who learned English as their first language may be enrolled in Native-language immersion program to learn the Native language as a second language. Native-language immersion involves students learning school subjects (math, science, social studies, music, and art) in the Native language for the whole day or most of the day. Successful Native-language immersion education programs systematically incorporate Native cultural content and culturally appropriate ways of teaching and learning. Three decades of research on Indigenous education in a range of contexts indicate that well-implemented Native-language immersion programs promote students' language acquisition and increase test performance, school retention, graduation rates, and college admission (McCarty, 2014).

Bilingual education has been shown to be beneficial for immigrant and refugee students as well. A large-scale study by Ramírez, Pasta, Yuen, Billings, and Ramey (1991), for instance, compared the academic performance of 2,352 Spanish-dominant Latino elementary schoolchildren in three types of classrooms: (1) English-only, (2) transitional bilingual, and (3) developmental bilingual. Ramírez et al. (1991) found that, although there were no differences among the program types in student achievement in third grade, students in developmental bilingual education programs were doing better in math, English language arts, and English reading than students in the other programs by sixth grade.

In another large-scale study involving 42,000 bilingual students in the United States, Thomas and Collier (2002) compared the scores on standardized tests of students enrolled in several types of programs. They found that programs that used students' home languages in education produced better results in English reading than programs that used only English. They also found that developmental and two-way immersion programs produced better results in English reading than transitional bilingual education programs.

Two-way immersion is a bilingual education model that typically involves about equal numbers of language-majority children and language-minority children learning both languages and school content in the same classroom. Each group serves as native-language models for the other group, and students learn each other's languages through social interaction. Similar to Thomas and Collier's (2002) findings, a review of research by Francis, Lesaux, and August (2006) revealed that language-minority students receiving instruction in both their native language and English did better on English reading assessments than language-minority students instructed only in English at both the elementary and secondary levels.

Findings like these may seem counterintuitive at first. Why would more schooling in the students' native language result in higher English scores? However, these findings make sense in light of the **linguistic interdependence principle**, the theory that first-language instruction not only develops native-language reading and writing skills but also language skills more generally in ways that support second language literacy (Cummins, 1996). Again, a bilingual's two languages are not separate compartments in the brain but are very much interconnected. For refugee-background adolescents with interrupted schooling or limited access to formal education, literacy instruction in a language that students understand is very important. These students often face the difficult task of acquiring literacy in a language they do not understand while simultaneously having to learn missed academic content. For this student population, multilingual approaches are crucial; attaining a foundation for literacy in their home language allows them to then transfer those skills to their second language.

Voices From the Classroom 10.1—Using First Language to Help With Vocabulary Acquisition

As an emergent bilingual teacher, I encounter many students who are strong in 1–2 components of language acquisition and struggle in other areas. Therefore, I make vocabulary exposure and word acquisition a priority, because I notice that when students are comfortable with basic reading comprehension, they become more comfortable using learned words in their conversations and in their writing. I encourage ELs to use their native language to support their English development by paying attention to cognates and emphasizing specific root and stem words, I highlight similarities and tell students that they often know more words than they think they do. I've noticed improvement when students realize that a word they already had in their language inventory can be used with minimal adaptation in their second language.

Gabriela Melendez, High School Bilingual Teacher

Bilingual education is not just for students that speak a minority language. For language-majority students, immersion education has been shown to lead to high levels of bilingualism and academic success. By far the most well-known and well-studied example is the case of French immersion in Canada. These early programs provided French-immersion education for English speakers in Quebec. The outcomes of the early immersion—consistent with findings from elsewhere in Canada—were often summarized as "two for one". That is, students achieved both a high level of second-language competence in French and mastery of academic content (e.g., math, social studies) similar to that of students studying through English, with no negative impacts on their English. These very positive findings deeply influenced education policy worldwide, with immersion programs developed in other countries such as Australia (in French, German, and Hebrew) and in Germany (in English, French, and Hungarian) among others.

While research has demonstrated clear potential of bilingual education for different populations across a range of contexts (e.g., Koh, Chen, Cummins, & Li, 2017), the unfortunate fact is that most students do not have the opportunity to take part in such programs. This is because, in many parts of the world, school is viewed as largely a monolingual space, where students are expected to acquire and function in the language of the society.

10.5 Helping Students Become Bilingual

Given this reality, how can we help more students to become bilingual? Educators who are committed to increasing bilingualism should understand that language majority speakers and language minority speakers have different needs when it comes to bilingual development. In order to become bilingual, majority language speakers need to have substantial opportunities to hear and speak the target language. It is simply not enough to have foreign language lessons for half an hour a day. Opportunity to study content material (e.g., math, science, social studies) through a target language offers both academic and linguistic benefits, with the potential to produce additive bilingualism.

For minority language speakers, however, because they are more susceptible to subtractive bilingualism, effective programs must go out of their way to prop up the weaker language. Thus, bilingual education programs for language minority students may actually deliver instruction in the minority language for some time so that students can develop a solid footing in that language before they are introduced to literacy in the majority language. These programs may provide continuous support in the students' native language even after students become proficient in the majority language, so they do not lose it. Although helping language minority students achieve additive bilingualism in the face of widespread monolingual bias may seem like a tall order, it is very possible with thoughtful planning and implementation.

As with all types of education, it is important to remember that there are no quick fixes, no one-size-fits-all models in bilingual education. A program that works well for a given student population may not work well with another group. Teachers, parents, and policy makers should study and learn from good practices but implementation of a successful bilingual education program will invariably require adapting the models to suit the needs of the local population. Ensuring successful bilingual education is perhaps more complex than monolingual education but the resulting gain for individuals and societies makes the effort worthwhile.

Further Reading

Howard, E. R., Sugarman, J., Christian, D., Lindholm-Leary, K. J., & Rogers, D. (2007). *Guiding principles for dual language education* (2nd ed.). Washington, DC: Center for Applied Linguistics.
Shin, S. J. (2018). *Bilingualism in schools and society: Language, identity, and policy* (2nd ed.). New York and London: Routledge.
Soltero, S. W. (2016). *Dual language education: Program design and implementation.* Portsmouth, NH: Heinemann.

Exercises

1. Do you consider yourself a bilingual? If so, what criteria did you use to determine that? How would you rate the level of your speaking, listening, reading, and writing skills in each language? Make a list of when you use each language and with whom. Has your ability in the languages changed over time? If so, what brought about those changes? If you do not consider yourself a bilingual, have you studied another language? How would you rate your proficiency in that language? What would it take for you to consider yourself bilingual in that language?
2. What is a deficit-based view of bilingualism? Why should educators be wary of labeling someone as "semilingual"? What are some ways in which teachers can promote additive bilingualism for majority-language-speaking students and for minority-language-speaking students?
3. Why is it harmful to advise immigrant and minority-language-speaking parents to speak the societal language with their children at home? What costs are incurred when parents and children cannot talk to each other due to a language barrier?
4. What factors contribute to making strong forms of bilingual education successful? What do they offer that are lacking in the weak forms of bilingual education?

References

Barac, R., Bialystok, E., Castro, D. C., & Sanchez, M. (2014). The cognitive development of young dual language learners: A critical review. *Early Childhood Research Quarterly, 29*(4), 699–714.

Bialystok, E., Luk, G., Peets, K. F., & Yang, S. (2010). Receptive vocabulary differences in monolingual and bilingual children. *Bilingualism: Language and Cognition, 13*(4), 525–531.

Chomsky, N. (1965). *Aspects of the theory of syntax*. Cambridge, MA: MIT Press.

Cummins, J. (1996). *Negotiating identities: Education for empowerment in a diverse society*. Ontario, CA: California Association for Bilingual Education.

Francis, D. J., Lesaux, N. K., & August, D. L. (2006). Language of instruction for language minority learners. In D. L. August & T. Shanahan (Eds.), *Developing literacy in second language learners: Report of the national literacy panel for language-minority children and youth* (pp. 365–414). Mahwah, NJ: Lawrence Erlbaum.

Klaus, D. (2003). The use of indigenous languages in early basic education in Papua New Guinea: A model for elsewhere? *Language and Education, 17*(2), 105–111.

Koh, P. W., Chen, X., Cummins, J., & Li, J. (2017). Literacy outcomes of a Chinese/English bilingual program in Ontario. *Canadian Modern Language Review, 73*(3), 343–367.

Lee, J. S. (2004). Linguistic hybridization in K-pop: Self-assertion and resistance. *World Englishes, 23*(3), 429–450.

McCarty, T. (2014). Teaching the whole child: Language immersion and student achievement. *Indian Country Today*. Retrieved July 26, 2017, from https://indiancountrymedianetwork.com/education/native-education/teaching-the-wholechild- language-immersion-and-student-achievement

Ramírez, D. J., Pasta, D. J., Yuen, S. D., Billings, D. K., & Ramey, D. R. (1991). *Longitudinal study of structured-English immersion strategy, early-exit, and late-exit transitional bilingual education programs for language minority children* (Vol. 2). San Mateo, CA: Aguirre International.

Thomas, W., & Collier, V. (2002). *A national study of school effectiveness for language minority students' long-term academic achievement*. Berkeley, CA: University of California Center for Research on Education, Diversity and Excellence.

UNESCO. (1953). *The use of vernacular languages in education*. Paris, France: UNESCO.

U.S. Census Bureau. (2015). *American community survey*. Detailed Languages Spoken at Home and Ability to Speak English for the Population 5 Years and Over for United States: 2009–2013. Retrieved August 27, 2017 from www.census.gov/data/tables/2013/demo/2009-2013-lang-tables.html

Valadez, C. M., MacSwan, J., & Martínez, C. (2000). Toward a new view of low-achieving bilinguals: A study of linguistic competence in designated "semilinguals". *Bilingual Review, 25*(3), 238–248.

11 Writing Systems

11.1 Introduction

Look around your surroundings right now. Chances are, you will see many examples of writing. Books and academic texts are good examples, certainly, but you might also notice writing on ordinary everyday things: labels, logos, notes, junk mail, takeout menus, posters, tags, bills, signs, websites, or today's date and time on your phone. Written language is an essential part of our daily lives, and this extends beyond the formal genre of academic texts and into informal registers. We use writing to send messages and exchange information. We use writing to tell stories and remember our history. We use writing to relate to others and learn about their lives.

It is important to look at all the different types of written language to better understand where our students are coming from, and what difficulties they might encounter when learning the written component of the target language. In this chapter, we first discuss the difference between written language and spoken language. We then describe how different types of writing systems have developed from earliest times. We explain how all writing can be grouped into two basic types—logographic (e.g., cuneiform, hieroglyphs, Chinese characters) and phonographic (e.g., syllabic writing, alphabetic writing). We will see that just as spoken language exhibits an arbitrary connection between sound and meaning, written language involves an arbitrary link between sound and symbol. Finally, we will discuss transparent versus opaque orthographies and the different literacy demands placed on readers of different languages.

11.2 Written Language vs. Spoken Language

In language teaching, we often talk about the four domains of language: listening, speaking, reading, and writing (see Table 11.1). However, what we don't often discuss as language teachers is how very different the first two domains—listening and speaking—are from the written domains, reading and writing. If you have tried to learn a second language, you might find that your oral language skills are at a different level than your written language skills. Some learners, like heritage speakers, tend to be more comfortable

Table 11.1 Domains of Language

	Receptive	Productive
Oral	Listening	Speaking
Written	Reading	Writing

with conversational spoken language but find written language more difficult. Meanwhile, other learners—like adult ESL students—find that they are much more comfortable with reading and writing but struggle with speaking and listening. You might also find that your students display a mismatch of skill level between their oral and written skills.

Why is this the case? Aren't all these skills just part of language? It turns out that although both oral and written skills are essential for academic success, there are some key differences. Firstly, spoken language has been around for over 100,000 years, but the earliest writing we have discovered goes back to only 3500 BC. This means that humans existed for over 95 millennia without written language. In comparison to spoken language, the written form is a very recent human invention.

Secondly, there are many cultures and languages that do not have an **orthography**, or written component. In fact, nearly half of the world's languages do not have an orthography. It is important to note that the lack of a writing system does not mean that a language is any less complex than those that are written. These cultures might have an oral tradition instead of a written tradition, and value other forms of record-keeping, storytelling, and communication that are not based on writing. Although knowing how to read and write is considered a necessity in many western cultures, this is not the case across all cultures.

Thirdly, spoken language and written language are different in that while babies do not need to be explicitly taught a first language—no one sits down an infant to teach them the alveolar fricative or verb conjugations—people do need to be explicitly taught how to read and write. A baby will acquire the spoken language without special instruction, but that same baby will not just naturally develop literacy skills by being next to a book. Literacy, or the ability to read and write, is very much an outcome of schooling.

Finally, one of the major differences between oral language and written language is that the former is an unedited, raw form of language that contains hesitations, false starts, and repetitions. Written language, however, is a processed, edited, and modifiable form of language. You can think about what you want to write before you write it, and usually you can edit what has been written to "clean it up", like you might do if you are constructing an email to your boss. You cannot really do that in spoken language: once it is spoken, it is out there. With written language you can read something over and over again, or you can read something slowly at your own pace. With listening, that is usually not possible unless it is a recording. In sum, oral language and written language are related but fundamentally quite different.

Voices From the Classroom 11.1—Differentiating Spoken and Written Language

To create a positive learning environment right from the start of the year in my World Language classroom, I found it particularly effective to take a moment to explain to my students how spoken language and written language are historically, structurally, and fundamentally very different from one another. I want them to know that, unlike written language, everyday spoken language is rarely perfect, even among native speakers, because it is not planned, revised, rehearsed, etc. I also make this same distinction with formal speeches, which while spoken, are written down, edited, rehearsed, and sometimes given with the aid of a teleprompter. Therefore, they should not expect their speaking skills in the target language to be perfect. The point here is, do not be afraid to make mistakes because everyone makes them! It's a natural part of spoken language and of the learning process.

Craig Boxx, High School World Language Teacher

11.3 Writing Systems

You are probably well aware there are many different types of writing systems in the world. You probably have come across Chinese characters before, used a few Greek letters in math or science, and have seen pictures of Egyptian hieroglyphs. What you may not have known is that a given alphabet can be used as writing systems for different languages. Take the Latin alphabet, for example. It is used to represent English, Spanish, French, Dutch, Icelandic, Croatian, Hungarian, and dozens of other European languages. Likewise, Chinese characters are used to represent various Chinese languages as well, like Mandarin, Cantonese, Hakka, and Taiwanese. Some languages like Azerbaijani, Turkmen, and Uzbek are officially in Latin but have a considerable number of users also writing them in Cyrillic.

American Sign Language (ASL) presents a very interesting case when it comes to writing. ASL users typically write in English. What is unique about this is that ASL speakers have to learn to read and write in a language that they do not hear, a remarkable feat given that ASL and English have vastly different syntactic structures. The takeaway from this is that writing systems are not dependent on the spoken—or signed—language itself. The relationship between a language and its writing system is quite arbitrary.

As spoken languages in contact borrow words and phrases from one another, scripts are often borrowed from one language to another, and some are developed out of a merge between two different writing systems. Written systems can also be related to one another the way that spoken languages can be. For example, the Tibetan writing system (Figure 11.1) was originally based on Sanskrit (Figure 11.2). The two share similar characteristics, most noticeable in the angular and downstroke lines.

གསུང་དང་སྦ་མ་རྣམས་ལ་ཕྱག་འཚལ་ལོ ॥

རྗེ་འགྲོ་བ་མགོན་པོ་དེ་བཞིན་ལ་འདུད ॥

སྦ་མ་མི་འགྱུར་ཚོས་ཀྱི་དང་ལ་བཤུགས ॥

ཕུན་རས་གཅིགས་ཀྱང་ཚོས་ཀྱི་དང་ལ་བཅུ ॥

ཕུ་རྗེ་ཆེན་པོ་ཚོས་ཀྱི་དང་ལ་བཤུགས ॥

ཕང་སྐྱོང་རྒྱལ་པོ་ཚོས་ཀྱི་དང་ལ་བཤུགས ॥

ཡོ་ཆེན་གོང་མ་ཚོས་ཀྱི་དང་ལ་བཤུགས ॥

ཀྲུ་སྟེ་ཁྲོམ་པ་ཨེག་དྲག་མ་རྗེ་རྡོངས ॥

ཨོཾ་མ་ཎི་པདྨེ་ཧཱུྃ །

Figure 11.1 Tibetan Script

अस्ति हस्तिनापुरे कर्पूरविलासो नाम रजकः । तस्य गर्द-
भो ऽतिभारवाहनादुर्बलो मुमूर्षुरिवाभवत् । ततस्तेन रज-
केनासौ व्याघ्रचर्मणा प्रच्छाद्यारण्यसमीपे सस्यक्षेत्रे मोचितः ।
ततो दूरादवलोक्य व्याघ्रबुद्ध्या क्षेत्रपतयः सर्वं पलायन्ते । स
च सुखेन सस्यं चरति । अथैकदा केनापि सस्यरक्षकेण धूसर-
कम्बलकृततनुत्राणेन धनुष्कारं सज्जीकृत्यावनतकायेनैकान्ते
स्थितम् । तं च दूरे दृष्ट्वा गर्दभः पुष्टाङ्गो गर्दभीयमिति मत्वा
शब्दं कुर्वाणस्तदभिमुखं धावितः । ततस्तेन सस्यरक्षकेण गर्द-
भो ऽयमिति ज्ञात्वा लीलयैव व्यापादितः ।

Figure 11.2 Sanskrit Script

All writing systems can be grouped into two main types: logographic and phonographic. Next we will discuss the characteristics of each type, as well as some examples of languages that use each system.

11.3.1 Logographic Systems

Logographic writing systems are orthographies in which symbols represent meanings. There is very little sound-to-symbol correspondence, such that learners would not be able to "sound things out" if they come across symbols they do not know. Each symbol and its associated meaning and sound must be learned individually and committed to memory. Logographic writing systems are among the earliest writing that have been discovered. The first known example is cuneiform, which was developed by the Sumerians around 3300 BC. As you can see in Figure 11.3, cuneiform is characterized by wedge-shaped cuts, which were carved into clay by a stylus. There were about 1000 different characters that were used in various combinations to express meaning. Another ancient form of writing is hieroglyphs, which were developed by Egyptians around 3000 BC. Hieroglyphs consist of **logograms** (symbols that represent meaning), **phonograms** (symbols that represent sound), and

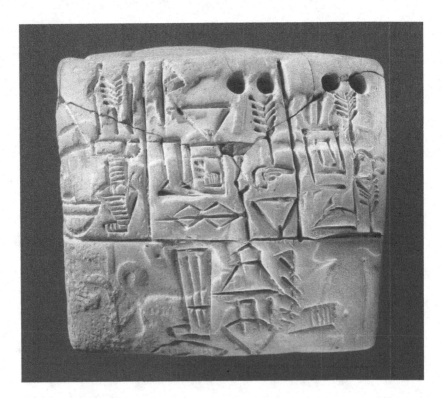

Figure 11.3 Sumerian Cuneiform

symbols that represent functional morphemes, such as plurality. Like cuneiform, hieroglyphs consist of about 1000 characters and are used in combination to represent language in written form.

Mayan glyphs are another example of a logographic writing system. These were developed around 300 BC in the Yucatán Peninsula of Mexico and are one of most complex writing systems discovered (Figure 11.4). Linguists have found that Mayan glyphs are comprised not only of logograms, but also of **rebus** symbols, which are pictorial representations of words. The Mayan writing system is so complex that scholars have only deciphered 85% of the glyphs to date (Katzner, 2002).

Another logographic writing system that people still use today is Chinese characters. Developed around 1200 BC in China, this system was historically used to represent languages such as Korean, Japanese, and Vietnamese. In present day, Chinese characters are used to represent Chinese languages such as Mandarin, Cantonese, and Shanghainese. In fact, even though many Chinese languages are mutually unintelligible, because they share a common writing system, speakers of different Chinese languages are able to communicate with one another through writing.

The Chinese writing system is composed of **radicals**, which are symbols that are combined to form a character. Chinese characters have both a meaning component and a pronunciation component. Examine the characters in Table 11.2. Notice that the radicals in the first column provide the meaning. The radicals in the second column provide the sound. In the last column are characters that combine both the meaning and sound components to give the reader information on the meaning and pronunciation of a character. For instance, in the first row, you will see that the radical for "water" is combined with that for "sheep" to form the character 洋 for "ocean". The radical for "water" 氵 provides the meaning component, and the phonogram 羊 provides the pronunciation component. Thus, you know that 洋 has a meaning related to water but pronunciation related to "yang". The same holds true for the rest of the examples.

Logographic writing systems are different from, say, a series of pictures that tell a story. In other words, logographic writing is not iconic. **Iconic** means that a symbol looks like its meaning, like a picture of a mountain to mean "mountain". Although logographic languages such as Chinese do have few iconic elements (e.g., 火 *huǒ* means "fire"; 山 *shān* means "mountain"), for the most part, logographic writing systems use an arbitrary system with no apparent connection between the meaning and its orthographic representation. In other words, the reader and writer have to know that the Chinese character 言 means "to speak", as there is nothing inherent about the shape of that character that lends itself to the meaning.

11.3.2 Phonographic Systems

Phonographic writing systems are those in which the symbols represent sounds. Languages that use a phonographic writing system allow readers to

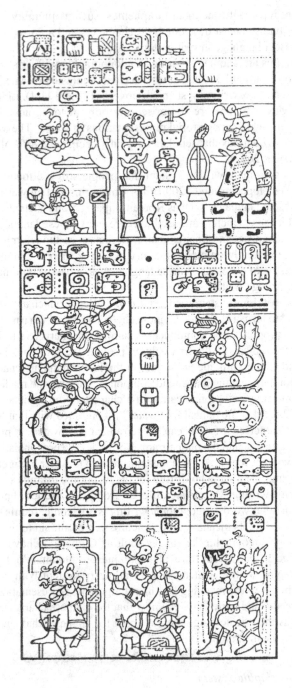

Figure 11.4 Mayan Glyphs

Table 11.2 Chinese Characters

Meaning	Pronunciation	Combined Character
氵 "water"	羊 "sheep" pronounced as \<yang\>	洋 "ocean" pronounced \<yang\>
氵 "water"	青 "green" pronounced as \<qing\>	清 "clear" pronounced as \<qing\>
氵 "water"	包 "bundle" pronounced as \<bao\>	泡 "soak" pronounced as \<bao\>
忄 "heart"	青 "green" pronounced as \<qing\>	情 "emotion" pronounced as \<qing\>
言 "word"	青 "green" pronounced as \<qing\>	請 "please" pronounced as \<qing\>

Table 11.3 Hiragana and Katakana

Phonetic	a	ka	sa	ta	na	ha	ma	ya	ra	wa	n
Sign	あ	か	さ	た	な	は	ま	や	ら	わ	ん
Hiragana Katakana	ア	カ	サ	タ	ナ	ハ	マ	ヤ	ラ	ワ	ン

Phonetic	i	ki	shi	chi	ni	hi	mi		ri		
Sign	い	き	し	ち	に	ひ	み		り		
Hiragana Katakana	イ	キ	シ	チ	ニ	ヒ	ミ		リ		

Phonetic	u	ku	su	tsu	nu	fu	mu	yu	ru		
Sign	う	く	す	つ	ぬ	ふ	む	ゆ	る		
Hiragana Katakana	ウ	ク	ス	ツ	ヌ	フ	ム	ユ	ル		

Phonetic	e	ke	se	te	ne	he	me		re		
Sign	え	け	せ	て	ね	へ	め		れ		
Hiragana Katakana	エ	ケ	セ	テ	ネ	ヘ	メ		レ		

Phonetic	o	ko	so	to	no	ho	mo	yo	ro	o	
Sign	お	こ	そ	と	の	ほ	も	よ	ろ	を	
Hiragana Katakana	オ	コ	ソ	ト	ノ	ホ	モ	ヨ	ロ	ヲ	

sound out a word because the way it is written is a direct clue as to how it is pronounced. The earliest known phonographic system was developed by the Phoenicians around 1500 BC. The alphabet consisted of 22 letters, all consonants and no vowels. The Phoenician alphabet is said to be the precursor to Greek and Latin alphabets. One type of phonographic writing system is syllabic writing system. In a **syllabic writing system**, characters represent syllables and are combined to form *morphemes*. Most commonly, syllabic writing systems only allow vowel (V) or consonant-vowel (CV) syllable structure. The Japanese kana (both hiragana and katakana—see Table 11.3) and Devanagari are examples of syllabic writing systems.

Another type of phonographic writing system is **alphabetic syllabary**, in which symbols that represent consonants and vowels are combined to form discrete phonograms, each representing one syllable. The Korean writing system, developed in the 15th century, is an example of alphabetic syllabary. The system has nineteen consonant symbols and twenty-one vowel symbols, each corresponding with a sound in the spoken language. The consonants and vowels are combined to form a phonogram representing one syllable. For instance, the Korean word for "mountain" is [san], which consists of one syllable made up of the sounds [s], [a], and [n]. The Korean letters ㅅ, ㅏ, ㄴ, corresponding to the sound [s], [a], and [n] respectively, are combined in a block to form the word 산. The onset is written in the upper left of the phonogram, the nucleus is written in the upper right of the phonogram, and the coda is written at the bottom of the phonogram. An example of a two-syllable word is the Korean word for "ocean", or [bada]. Since there are two syllables in [bada], there are two phonograms, one for [ba] and one for [da]. The Korean letters ㅂ, ㅏ, ㄷ, ㅏ correspond to the sounds [b], [a], [d], [a], respectively, and are combined to form the two phonograms, 바다. Since neither syllable has a coda, the bottom slot of the phonogram is empty.

Another type of phonographic writing system is the one you are using to read right now: **alphabetic writing**. Alphabetic writing systems have symbols corresponding to sounds in the language it represents, and these symbols are strung together in sequence to form morphemes, words, and phrases. These symbols can be written and read from left to right or right to left. Some alphabetic writing systems are consonantal systems, in which the writing supplies the consonants and the reader must fill in the vowels as they read. For example, the Arabic writing system, developed around 700, is used to represent many spoken languages today including Arabic, Persian, Urdu, and Pashto. The Arabic alphabet has twenty-eight consonants and is written from right to left. Although there are a few symbols for vowels, the writing is largely consonantal, and readers can easily figure out what the words mean through context. For example, the word for "child" in Arabic is [tˤifl]. Although the spoken pronunciation has the vowel [i], only the consonants [tˤ] ط, [f] ف and [l] ل are written: طفل.

11.4 Learning to Read and Write

Earlier, we talked about how reading and writing are very different from speaking and listening. Reading and writing require explicit instruction, meaning you cannot just pick them up by watching someone read or being next to someone who is writing. Although written language is a representation of spoken language, the connection between the two is largely arbitrary. In other words, there is really no particular rationale between how something is said and how something is written. For instance, the English word "cat" is pronounced [kæt]. But there is nothing about a voiceless velar stop, a low front vowel, and a voiceless alveolar stop that look anything like the letters *c*, *a*, and *t*. For all it matters, it could be written as ♏︎♋︎♦ or □. The point is, there is no logical connection between sound and symbol; the relationship is completely arbitrary.

Perhaps this is one of the reasons why learning to read and write takes time for learners. Even native speakers, who have been exposed to the spoken language from birth, do not naturally and spontaneously learn to read and write. As we said before, left alone, native speakers would become fine speakers of the language but would be illiterate. Similarly, we cannot expect a second language learner to just spontaneously learn to read and write, even if their first language has a similar writing system. Heritage speakers, who grow up speaking a language at home that is different from the one they use at school or society, might have excellent speaking and listening skills but struggle with reading or writing because they have not been taught it. Relatedly, just because a student can speak well does not necessarily mean they can read and write at the same level.

Difficulty with reading and writing may be linked to how closely and consistently a sound corresponds to a symbol. Yes, the logical connection between sound and symbol is almost always arbitrary, but the *correspondence* between sound and symbol can differ. In other words, there is a range when it comes to sound-to-symbol correspondence. Let us give you an example. Suppose Language A contains the sound [s] in its phonetic inventory, and the written language represents it as ◆. Every time a word contains the [s] sound, whether at the beginning, middle, or end of the word, it is always represented as ◆ in writing. That means Language A has close sound-to-symbol correspondence. This makes things easy; you know that every time you see ◆ in writing, it will always be pronounced [s]. Now, let us suppose Language B contains the sound [s], but it is sometimes represented as ❀, other times it appears as ❖, and in some cases it can be written as ■. A language like Language B has a less direct and correspondence between sound and symbol. This is a little more difficult for learners because it is less consistent.

Writing systems that have a close sound-to-symbol correspondence are said to have a **shallow (transparent) orthography**. These systems have a more consistent 1:1 correspondence between the sound and symbol, such that whenever a reader sees a particular symbol, they know it will always make one particular sound. Languages like Spanish, Italian, and Korean have transparent orthographies. Students who study these languages learn the orthographies faster because of the consistency. They also tend to have better accuracy when reading aloud as a result. In fact, even if you have not studied Italian, if you were given a passage in Italian, you could probably read it aloud right now with decent accuracy. Of course, you wouldn't know the meaning of what you read, but you could sound out most words. A quick five-minute primer on how to decipher the more difficult aspects of Italian orthography (e.g., *ch* is pronounced [k]) would probably boost your accuracy significantly.

Let us take Spanish as another example. Whenever the letter *e* appears in Spanish writing, it is always pronounced the same way, [e]. Whether the *e* appears at the beginning, end, or middle of a word, and whether it comes before or after certain combinations of letters, it will always be pronounced

[e]. For example, the *e* in all these words is pronounced the same way: *b<u>e</u>so* "kiss", *<u>e</u>ntre* "between", *call<u>e</u>* "street", *tr<u>e</u>inta* "thirty". The point is, the closer the sound-to-symbol correspondence, the easier it is to learn to read and write in that language.

In contrast, there is less direct correspondence between sounds and symbols in languages that have **deep (opaque) orthographies**. Languages like French and English have opaque orthographies. Think about all the ways we can represent the schwa vowel [ə] in English: *<u>a</u>live, r<u>e</u>pair, d<u>i</u>rect, p<u>o</u>lite, <u>u</u>ndo, c<u>ou</u>sin*. For the single sound, there are a handful of different ways it can be written. This goes the other way as well. The same letter can have multiple pronunciations: *c* can be pronounced two different ways, (*<u>c</u>ake, la<u>c</u>e* as [k] and [s], respectively); *gh* can have three different pronunciations (*rou<u>gh</u>, <u>gh</u>ost, thou<u>gh</u>* as [f], [g], and ø respectively); *ea* can be pronounced three ways (*<u>ea</u>ch, br<u>ea</u>d, gr<u>ea</u>t* as [i], [ɛ], [ei]). Languages with logographic writing systems are all opaque, as there is very little sound-to-symbol correspondence by design. Learners of Chinese, for example, must learn the characters that represent meaning, sound, and morphology, and have to combine these elements to write.

Students who learn opaque orthographies tend to take longer to learn how to read and write. This includes native-speaking children; it might take children several years to fully learn to decode a language they already speak. The added difficulty for second language learners, of course, is that they have to learn to read and write at the same time that they are learning to speak and listen. In both native and nonnative cases, students cannot always rely on sounding words out, so words must be learned by sight. These are what are known as **sight words**, or words that have to be memorized visually in chunks because they do not follow the standard rules of pronunciation. Some early sight words that are taught to English-speaking children include the following: *the, their, there, he, she, these, would, could, because, right*.

Students sometimes struggle when learning to read and write in their second language because they come from a system that functions quite differently. For instance, if English speakers are learning Greek, they have to learn a new phonetic alphabet. But sometimes the writing systems can differ in more ways than just the symbols. For instance, if you have students who are used to a phonographic alphabet in their first language (English) and are learning a logographic system (Chinese), they have to understand that a single character can combine not only sound but also meaning. Even more challenging is when the script looks the same, but the conventions are different. For example, Spanish speakers are used to a script that is quite transparent, with consistent sound-to-symbol correspondence. However, when they learn English, they may be lulled into a false sense of security because the script looks the same—Spanish and English writing systems both use the same alphabet—but one is a transparent system and other is an opaque system. Spanish speakers can no longer rely on the fact that an *e* is always pronounced like [e]; it can be pronounced as [ɛ], [i], [ə], or silent: *b<u>e</u>d, m<u>e</u>, <u>e</u>lect, mic<u>e</u>*.

Voices From the Classroom 11.2—Helping Spanish Speakers Learn English Spelling

I have observed that some Spanish-speaking children who are used to spelling easily in Spanish are disappointed to find it difficult to spell in English. But when they phoneticize the English word in the same way they learned to do in Spanish, then it no longer is a problem. For example, the children take the word *beautiful* and sound it out in Spanish: *bĕ, ah, oo, tĭ, fōōl*. Then they write the word as they hear it in Spanish. This way they can remember all the vowels in the English word.

From: Igoa, C. (1995). *The Inner World of the Immigrant Child*. Mahwah, NJ: Erlbaum.

In sum, it is important for language teachers to be aware of three main facts. Firstly, we must keep in mind that there is a disconnect between the oral language and written language, and students may show higher proficiency with one but not the other. This is not because there is a problem with the student necessarily, but because oral and written language are related but separate skills. Teachers are sometimes puzzled when their excellent speaker has difficulty writing an essay in the same language, but this is like expecting an excellent piano player to just naturally play the guitar well too. Secondly, it is crucial to keep in mind that there is a wide range of differences between writing systems, with some that use symbols to represent sound and others that use symbols to represent both meaning and sound. Switching one's mindset from one system to another is not an automatic process. Lastly, it is important to remember that even among writing systems that are similar, like English and Spanish, there are differences in the sound-to-symbol correspondence that can make reading and writing difficult. The superficial similarity can be misleading and deceptively difficult if one is transparent and the other is opaque.

Further Reading

Crystal, D. (2010). *The Cambridge encyclopedia of language* (3rd ed.). Cambridge, UK: Cambridge University Press.
Daniels, P. T., & Bright, W. (Eds.). (1996). *The world's writing systems*. New York: Oxford University Press.
Katzner, K. (2002). *The languages of the world* (3rd ed.). New York: Routledge.

Exercises

1. Writing and speaking are fundamentally different. Record someone speaking spontaneously for one minute and transcribe it. Note how the spoken language is different from written language.

2. Rebus puzzles are word picture puzzles with hidden meanings. Two examples of a rebus puzzle are seen below:

   STAN4CE   ("4 in stance" → "For instance")

   MIND
   MATTER   ("mind over matter")

   You can also find many examples of rebus puzzles online.

   a. What are the characteristics of rebus puzzles? How do they relate to both logographic and phonographic systems?
   b. Construct two rebus puzzles of your own. How might these help learners with both meaning and pronunciation?

3. Unlike spoken language, written language is a human construction. Design your own writing system to represent a language that you speak. Choose a logographic system or phonographic system. What are some considerations you have to consider? Challenges?

4. Look at the following groups of sight words in English. What makes these difficult to sound out? What are some of the incongruities in the sound-to-symbol correspondence in each group?

   a. think, the
   b. some, sum
   c. though, through, thought
   d. read (present tense), read (past tense)
   e. said, paid
   f. why, what, who

References

Igoa, C. (1995). *The inner world of the immigrant child*. Mahwah, NJ: Erlbaum
Katzner, K. (2002). *The languages of the world* (3rd ed.). New York: Routledge.

Glossary

accent   The phonological patterning of a language or dialect

additive bilingualism   A situation in which one learns a second language while continuing to use the first language

adjectives   Open class words whose key function is to modify nouns

adverbs   Open class words that modify verbs, adjectives, prepositions, and other adverbs

affix   A morpheme that is attached to the beginning, end, middle, or around a root to change its meaning or function

affricates   Sounds produced by a stop closure followed immediately by a slight release of the articulators so that turbulent noise is produced

African American English   A fully-fledged language spoken primarily by African Americans in the U.S.

allomorphs   The alternate phonetic forms of a morpheme

allophones   Predictable variants of one phoneme

alphabetic writing   Orthographies in which symbols that represent sounds are written linearly to form a sequence of sounds

alveolar ridge   The small ridge in the mouth just behind the upper teeth

alveolars   Sounds produced by raising the front part of the tongue to the alveolar ridge

alveopalatals   Sounds produced by raising the front part of the tongue to a point on the hard palate just behind the alveolar ridge. See also **post-alveolars**

antonyms   Words that have opposite meanings

articulators   The principal parts of the vocal tract that can be used to make sounds

aspirated   Sounds that are produced with a significant puff of air

assimilation   A phonological process in which a sound becomes more like a neighboring sound in terms of one or more of its phonetic characteristics

auxiliaries   Closed class words that provide information such as conditionality, future expression, aspect, and mood

back   The back part of the tongue body

back vowels   Vowels produced with the tongue close to the back surface of the vocal tract

bilabials   Sounds produced by bringing the two lips together

blade   The area just behind the tip of the tongue

borrowing   An aspect of one language is permanently added to the linguistic repertoire of another language. See also **loan words**

bound morpheme   A morpheme that can only occur in words attached to other morphemes

case   A grammatical feature that indicates the function of a noun

center   The middle part of the tongue body

central vowels   Vowels produced with the tongue midway between the front and back of the mouth

chain shift   Changes in historical phonology in which one sound influences the change of another, forming a chain reaction

Chicano English   A fully-fledged language spoken primarily by Mexican-Americans in the U.S.

circumfixes   Affixes that are attached to the front and the end of the root to form new words

clause   Units of language (constituents) that are just above the level of phrases. Consists of a predicate and usually a subject

closed class   Class of words where adding new words to the categories are highly infrequent

coda   The part of the syllable following the nucleus, consists of one or more consonants

code-switching   The alternating use of two or more languages within the same conversation, usually when bilinguals are in the company of other bilinguals

cognates   Words that have the same linguistic derivation from the same original word or root

commissives   Speech acts that affect the speaker and commission oneself to a course of action

complementizers   Closed class words that connect clauses together

complex words   Words that contain two or more morphemes

compounding   The process of building a new word by combining two or more existing words.

conjunctions   Closed class words that join two words, phrases, or clauses of equal grammatical weight

consonant cluster reduction   A phenomenon in which consonant blends are simplified to a single consonant

constituency   The property in which a word or group of words form a single unit of language

constituents   A word or group of words that form a single unit of language

content morphemes   Morphemes that carry meaning as opposed to merely perform a grammatical function

contour tones   Shifts of pitch from one to another in tonal languages

cooperative principle   A principle which describes how people achieve effective conversational communication in social situations. Developed by Paul Grice

creaky voice See **vocal fry**

creole A newly formed language that has arisen out of a contact variety, usually from what used to be a pidgin

creolization The process by which a pidgin becomes a creole

daughter The node one level directly below

declaratives Speech acts that change the world around the speaker

deletion A phonological process in which a sound is eliminated

dependent clause Clause that is usually embedded in other sentences and begins with a complementizer. Also called **embedded clause**

derivational morphemes Morphemes that change either the meaning or the part of speech of the word

descriptive linguistics The objective, scientific study of language whose goal is to describe the language as it is used

determiners Closed class words that provide information such as definiteness, quantification, possession, or demonstrative

developmental bilingual education An educational model in which students are instructed in the native language to establish a strong foundation, and the majority language is gradually added to the program to promote additive bilingualism

devoicing A phonological process in which a voiced sound becomes voiceless

diacritic An additional symbol written above or below a letter or IPA symbol to indicate further pronunciation information

dialect A variety that has all the components and complexity of a language, but has less social power or prestige

diphthongs Vowels that move from one vowel to another; a sound formed by the combination of two vowels in a single syllable

directives Speech acts in which the speaker compels the listener to do something

dissimilation A phonological process in which a sound becomes less like a neighboring sound in terms of one of more of its phonetic characteristics

embedded clause See **dependent clause**

expanded pidgin In pidgin formation, where the pidgin expands its usage across different domains of life

expressives Speech acts in which the speaker expresses one's attitudes or state of affairs

false cognates Pairs of words that appear to be cognates because of similar sounds (and meaning) but in fact are not cognates because they have different origins

flapping A phonological process in which a sound becomes a flap or tap

fragment A clause that is missing a component or a dependent clause that is not embedded in an independent clause

free morpheme A morpheme that can stand alone as a word

fricatives Sounds produced when the airstream is partially obstructed to allow air to continuously flow through the mouth

front   The front part of the tongue body

front vowels   Vowels produced with the highest point of the tongue in the front of the mouth

function morphemes   Morphemes that provide information about the grammatical relationships between words in a sentence

gender   A grammatical feature that classifies nouns into different categories (such as masculine, feminine, neutral)

generative grammar   The recursive nature of language that allows infinite combinations of utterances from a small subset of rules

glides   Sounds produced as the vocal organs move toward or away from articulation of a vowel or consonant. See also **semivowels**

glottals   Sounds produced by using the vocal cords as primary articulators with no other modification of the airstream in the mouth

glottis   Area of the throat containing the vocal cords

Great Vowel Shift   A massive sound change that marked the transition from Middle English to Early Modern English

hard palate   The bony structure in the roof of the mouth

head   The mandatory and most important component of the phrase that gives the phrase its category

heritage language learners   Speakers that learned the target language primarily at home or in non-academic settings

high vowels   Vowels produced with the tongue raised high in the mouth

homophony   The phenomenon in which multiple words with different meanings have the same pronunciation

hyponym   Words with a specific meaning that falls under a general category or set

hypercorrection   Correcting oneself beyond what is necessary

hypernym   Superordinate word that forms a set or category in which other specific words fall under

iconic   Characteristic of writing in which a symbol looks like its meaning

independent clause   Clause that can stand alone, also called sentence

infix   An affix that is inserted into an existing morpheme

inflected   Containing one or more affix

inflection   A morphological process that changes the form of a word to express a grammatical function or attribute

inflection   A process of word formation, in which a word is modified to express different grammatical categories such as tense, case, voice, aspect, number, and gender

inflectional morphemes   Affixes that are added to a word to assign a specific grammatical property to that word

insertion   A phonological process in which a sound is added

interdentals   Sounds produced by inserting the tip of the tongue between the upper and lower teeth

internal modification   A morphological process that substitutes one sound for another to mark a grammatical contrast

intonation   Pitch movement that does not change the meaning of a word

intransitive   A type of predicate that disallows a direct object

jargon   Specialized vocabulary for a particular interest group

jargon stage   The stage of pidgin formation in which there is a small vocabulary that is limited to one specific purpose

L1   First language

L2   Second language

labiodentals   Sounds produced by touching the top teeth to the lower lip

lateral   Sound produced by releasing air around the sides of the tongue

lax vowels   Vowels produced with wider mouth opening and relaxed muscles in the vocal tract

length   The duration of a speech sound

lexical borrowing   Words and phrases that are borrowed from one language to another

lexical semantics   The study of how meaning is created within and between words

lexifier   In a language contact situation, the language that contributes the most vocabulary

lingua franca   A common language spoken between different language communities

linguistic competence   Subconscious knowledge of one's language that provides intuition about the well-formedness of the language

linguistic interdependence principle   The theory that first-language instruction not only develops native-language reading and writing skills but also language skills more generally in ways that support second language literacy

liquids   Sounds that involve substantial constriction of the vocal tract but the constriction is not sufficiently narrow to block the vocal tract or cause friction

loan words   Words that have been borrowed from other languages. See also **borrowing**

logographic   Orthographies in which symbols represent a meaning, whether that be a morpheme, word, or phrase

low vowels   Vowels produced with the tongue low in the mouth

Mainstream American English   The most commonly spoken variety of American English in the U.S.

manner assimilation   A phonological process in which the manner of articulation of a sound becomes more like the manner of articulation of a neighboring sound

manner of articulation   The way the airstream is modified by the articulators in the vocal tract to produce sounds

maxim of manner   A guideline for effective conversation that suggests one should be orderly and clear, and not be ambiguous

maxim of quality   A guideline for effective conversation that suggests one should be truthful

maxim of quantity   A guideline for effective conversation that suggests one should be as informative as required, but no more than is adequate

maxim of relevance   A guideline for effective conversation that suggests one should be as relevant as possible

metathesis   A phonological process that reorders sounds, often to make it easier to pronounce or understand

mid vowels   Vowels produced with the tongue at mid-level height in the mouth

Middle English   The period of English language history from c. 1150 to c. 1450

minimal pairs   Pairs of words in a language that differ by only one sound and result in a difference in meaning

minimal set   A set of words in a language that differ by only one sound and result in a difference in meaning

modals   A type of auxiliary that expresses modality, such as doubt, certainty, permission, ability, or obligation

Modern English   The period of English language history from c. 1450 to the present

morpheme   The smallest linguistic unit with a meaning or a grammatical function

morphology   The study of the internal structure and formation of words in language

mother   The node one level directly above

movement   A shuffling of the word order of sentences, such as to create a question or passive construction

nasal cavity   The inside of the nose

nasal sound   A sound created when the soft palate is lowered and air moves through the nose. See also **nasals**

nasal stops   Sounds produced when air is stopped in the oral cavity and escapes through the nose

nasals   Sounds produced by lowering the velum and opening the nasal passage to the vocal tract. See also **nasal sound**

natural class   A group of sounds in a language that share one or more articulatory or auditory property, to the exclusion of other sounds in that language

negative concord   A language characteristic in which two negative words still equal a negative meaning

negative polarity items   Negation words

node   A joint in a tree diagram

non-tonal languages   Languages in which pitch differences do not change the meaning of a word

nonstandard dialect   A dialect that lacks overt social prestige and status

Northern Cities Chain Shift   A prominent sound change currently ongoing in the upper Midwest region of the United States

nouns   Open class words that generally refer to people, places, events, things, or ideas

nucleus The vowel portion of a syllable

null copula A phenomenon in which the copula can be dropped in some grammatical cases. See also **zero copula**

null subject languages See **prodrop languages**

number A grammatical feature that expresses plurality

obligatory rules Phonological rules that apply in the speech of all speakers of a language or dialect having the rule, regardless of style or rate of speaking

obstruents A natural class of consonants made up of stops, fricatives, and affricates

Old English The period of English language history from c. 450 to c. 1150

onset The part of the syllable preceding the nucleus, consists of one or more consonants

opaque writing system Orthographies that have less direct correspondence between sounds and symbols. Also called **deep orthography**

open class Class of words where adding new words to the categories are highly frequent

optional rules Phonological rules that may or may not apply in any given utterance and are responsible for variation in speech

oral cavity The inside of the mouth

oral sound A sound created when the soft palate is raised and air moves through the mouth

oral stops Sounds produced when air is stopped in the nasal cavity and escapes through the mouth

orthography The writing system of a language

palatals Sounds produced with the tongue on or near the palate

palate The highest part of the roof of the mouth

paradigm leveling A phenomenon in which the irregular components of a grammatical or phonological paradigm becomes regularized, becoming more consistent with the rest of the paradigm

parts of speech The grouping of words into categories based on grammatical function

performative speech act Speech acts in which the words themselves are the action

person A grammatical feature that expresses information about the subject

pharynx A tube in the throat just above the vocal cords

phonemes Sounds in a given language that are heard by its native speakers as distinct sounds and that result in a difference in meaning when interchanged

phonetic inventory The set of sounds in a particular language

phonetics The study of sounds in language

phonographic Orthographies in which symbols represent sound and have high sound-to-symbol correspondence

phonology The study of sound patterns in language

phonotactic rules The language-specific constraints of what is or is not permissible for pronunciation in a language

phrasal semantics   The study of how meaning can be constructed and construed at the phrase or sentence level

phrase structure rules   Templates for each type of phrase, containing information about what constituents are allowed and in what position they may appear

phrases   Units of language (constituents) that are just above the level of words

pidgin   A limited communication tool used between different speech communities; not a language

pitch   The auditory property of a sound that can be placed on a scale that ranges from low to high

place assimilation   A phonological process in which the place of articulation of a sound becomes more like the place of articulation of a neighboring sound

place of articulation   The point where the airstream is obstructed to produce a different sound

polysemy   The phenomenon in which the same word has multiple different meanings

post-alveolars   See **alveopalatals**

pragmatics   The study of language use in context

predicate   The core element of the clause, often headed by a verb, that provides information about the clause's function and components

prefix   An affix that is attached to the front of the root

prepositions   Closed class words that indicate relationships in space and time

prescriptive linguistics   The subjective study of language whose goal is to prescribe how language should be used

primary stress   The most prominently stressed syllable in the word

prodrop languages   Languages that allow the subject (and/or object) pronouns to be omitted when understood by context. See also **subject drop** and **null subject languages**

radicals   Symbols that are combined to form a character

reduplication   A morphological process that changes a word's meaning by repeating or copying all or part of the word

reference   The relation between the linguistic expression and the existence of that entity in the real world

referent   A person or thing to which a linguistic expression refers

register tones   Level tones that describe specific points within a pitch range in tonal languages

representatives   Speech acts consisting of assertions or claims that the speaker believes to be true

retroflex   Sounds produced by curling the tip of the tongue back

rhyme   The part of the syllable containing the nucleus and coda

root   The part of the tongue that lies opposite the back wall of the pharynx; also the primary lexical unit of a word that carries the most significant aspects of semantic content and cannot be reduced into smaller parts

rounded vowels Vowels produced with lips in a circular position

run-on Two independent clauses in one sentence

secondary stress The second most prominently stressed syllable in a word

segments Consonants and vowels

semantic roles The functions that a predicate can assign to the various constituents around them. See also **thematic roles** or **theta roles**

semantics The study of meaning in language

semivowels See **glides**

sense The concept or mental representation of a word

sight words Words that have to be memorized visually as a whole because they do not follow the standard rules of decoding

simple words Words that are made up of a single morpheme

sister A node on the same level, shares a mother node

slang Words or phrases that are relatively new to the language, used in informal settings often to display in-group membership

soft palate See **velum**

speech acts Actions performed through language

speech community A group of people that share a common language or dialect

stabilized pidgin In pidgin formation, a more established and consistent set of words, phrases, and syntax for communication

standard dialect An agreed-upon variety of a language that is used across an area

stops Sounds produced when there is a complete closure of the articulators and air is stopped

strengthening A phonological process that makes sounds stronger

stress Syllable features that is typically longer, louder, and higher in pitch

stress-timed languages Languages where the stressed syllables are said at approximately regular intervals, and unstressed syllables shorten to fit the rhythm

strong form of bilingual education Form of bilingual education whose language outcome is bilingualism and biliteracy

structural borrowing Borrowing of entire structures that did not originally exist in the borrowing language and that end up becoming a permanent feature

subject The part of the clause outside of the predicate

subject drop See **prodrop languages**

substrate In a language contact situation, the language spoken by the less socially powerful people

subtractive bilingualism A situation in which the socially dominant language replaces the weaker minority language

suffix An affix that is attached to the end of the root

superstrate In a language contact situation, the language spoken by the people in power

suppletion A morphological process that marks a grammatical contrast by replacing a morpheme with a completely different morpheme

suprasegmentals   Speech features that are added over segments. Includes features such as pitch, stress, and length

syllabic writing   Orthographies in which symbols that represent sounds are combined to form discrete phonograms, each representing one syllable

syllable   A unit of pronunciation having one vowel sound, with or without surrounding consonants, forming the whole or a part of a word

syllable-timed languages   Languages in which every syllable is approximately the same length

synonyms   Words that are similar in meaning

syntax   The study of rules and principles of sentence structure in language

tense   A grammatical feature that expresses time

tense vowels   Vowels produced with narrower mouth opening and constricted muscles in the vocal tract

terminal node   An end node in a tree diagram that does not have further nodes branching off it

thematic roles   See **semantic roles**

theta roles   See **semantic roles**

tip   The narrow area at the front of the tongue

tonal languages   Languages in which pitch differences change the meaning of a word

tone   Pitch differences that change the meaning of a word

tongue   A fleshy muscular organ in the mouth that can produce fine and complex movements

tongue body   The main mass of the tongue

transitional bilingual education   An educational model in which students are provided native language instruction only as a temporary bridge to learning English or other majority language

transitive   A type of predicate that requires a direct object

transitivity   A property of predicates that determines whether or not it has a direct object

transparent writing system   Orthographies that have a close sound-to-symbol correspondence. Also called **shallow orthography**

tree diagram   A visual representation of the inner structure and hierarchies within phrases and clauses

trill   Sounds produced by the articulators vibrating

two-way immersion   Bilingual education model that typically involves about equal numbers of language-majority children and language-minority children learning both languages and school content in the same classroom

unaspirated   Sounds that are produced without a significant puff of air

unrounded vowels   Vowels produced with lips in a relaxed position

upspeak   The phenomenon in which declarative sentences end with a rising intonation. Also called **uptalk**

uptalk   See **upspeak**

uvula   A tear-shaped piece of soft tissue at the lower end of the soft palate

velars   Sounds produced with the tongue on or near the velum

velum   A muscular flap in the back of the mouth that can be raised to press against the back wall of the pharynx to prevent air from escaping through the nose. See also **soft palate**

verbs   Open class words that generally function as a key element of the predicate

vocal cords   Folds of tissue in the throat through which air passes to make sound

vocal fry   A deep, creaky tone of voice that is made by relaxing the vocal cords but expelling the same amount of air, resulting in a creaky tone. Also called **creaky voice**

vocal tract   The air passages above the larynx, including the oral cavity, the nasal cavity, and the pharynx

voiced   Sounds made when the vocal cords are vibrating

voiceless   Sounds made when the vocal cords are apart

voicing assimilation   A phonological process in which the voicing of a sound becomes more like the voicing of a neighboring sound

weak form of bilingual education   Form of bilingual education whose language outcome is monolingualism or limited bilingualism

weakening   A phonological process that makes sounds weaker

wh-word   Question words, including who, what, when, where, why, how, which

World Englishes   International varieties of English spoken in three circles: the inner circle, the outer circle, and the expanding circle

zero copula   See **null copula**

THE INTERNATIONAL PHONETIC ALPHABET (revised to 2018)

CONSONANTS (PULMONIC)

© 2018 IPA

	Bilabial	Labiodental	Dental	Alveolar	Postalveolar	Retroflex	Palatal	Velar	Uvular	Pharyngeal	Glottal
Plosive	p b			t d		ʈ ɖ	c ɟ	k g	q ɢ		ʔ
Nasal	m	ɱ		n		ɳ	ɲ	ŋ	N		
Trill	B			r					R		
Tap or Flap		ⱱ		ɾ		ɽ					
Fricative	ɸ β	f v	θ ð	s z	ʃ ʒ	ʂ ʐ	ç ʝ	x ɣ	χ ʁ	ħ ʕ	h ɦ
Lateral fricative				ɬ ɮ							
Approximant		ʋ		ɹ		ɻ	j	ɰ			
Lateral approximant				l		ɭ	ʎ	L			

Symbols to the right in a cell are voiced, to the left are voiceless. Shaded areas denote articulations judged impossible.

CONSONANTS (NON-PULMONIC)

Clicks	Voiced implosives	Ejectives
ʘ Bilabial	ɓ Bilabial	' Examples:
ǀ Dental	ɗ Dental/alveolar	p' Bilabial
ǃ (Post)alveolar	ʄ Palatal	t' Dental/alveolar
ǂ Palatoalveolar	ɠ Velar	k' Velar
ǁ Alveolar lateral	ʛ Uvular	s' Alveolar fricative

OTHER SYMBOLS

ʍ Voiceless labial-velar fricative

w Voiced labial-velar approximant

ɥ Voiced labial-palatal approximant

ʜ Voiceless epiglottal fricative

ʢ Voiced epiglottal fricative

ʡ Epiglottal plosive

ɕ ʑ Alveolo-palatal fricatives

ɺ Voiced alveolar lateral flap

ɧ Simultaneous ʃ and x

Affricates and double articulations can be represented by two symbols joined by a tie bar if necessary.

t͡s k͡p

VOWELS

Front   Central   Back

Close i•y ——— ɨ•ʉ ——— ɯ•u

I Y   ʊ

Close-mid e•ø ——— ɘ•ɵ ——— ɤ•o

ə

Open-mid ɛ•œ — ɜ•ɞ — ʌ•ɔ

æ   ɐ

Open a•ɶ ——— ɑ•ɒ

Where symbols appear in pairs, the one to the right represents a rounded vowel.

SUPRASEGMENTALS

ˈ Primary stress

ˌ Secondary stress

ˌfoʊnəˈtɪʃ

ː Long eː

ˑ Half-long eˑ

˘ Extra-short ĕ

| Minor (foot) group

‖ Major (intonation) group

. Syllable break ɹi.ækt

‿ Linking (absence of a break)

DIACRITICS Some diacritics may be placed above a symbol with a descender, e.g. ŋ̊

̥ Voiceless	n̥ d̥	̤ Breathy voiced	b̤ a̤	̪ Dental	t̪ d̪
̬ Voiced	s̬ t̬	̰ Creaky voiced	b̰ a̰	̺ Apical	t̺ d̺
ʰ Aspirated	tʰ dʰ	̼ Linguolabial	t̼ d̼	̻ Laminal	t̻ d̻
̹ More rounded	ɔ̹	ʷ Labialized	tʷ dʷ	̃ Nasalized	ẽ
̜ Less rounded	ɔ̜	ʲ Palatalized	tʲ dʲ	ⁿ Nasal release	dⁿ
̟ Advanced	u̟	ˠ Velarized	tˠ dˠ	ˡ Lateral release	dˡ
̠ Retracted	e̠	ˤ Pharyngealized	tˤ dˤ	̚ No audible release	d̚
̈ Centralized	ë	̴ Velarized or pharyngealized	ɫ		
̽ Mid-centralized	e̽	̝ Raised	e̝ (ɹ̝ = voiced alveolar fricative)		
̩ Syllabic	n̩	̞ Lowered	e̞ (β̞ = voiced bilabial approximant)		
̯ Non-syllabic	e̯	̘ Advanced Tongue Root	e̘		
˞ Rhoticity	ɚ a˞	̙ Retracted Tongue Root	e̙		

TONES AND WORD ACCENTS

LEVEL		CONTOUR	
e̋ or ˥	Extra high	ě or ˩˥	Rising
é or ˦	High	ê or ˥˩	Falling
ē or ˧	Mid	e᷄ or ˦˥	High rising
è or ˨	Low	e᷅ or ˩˨	Low rising
ȅ or ˩	Extra low	e᷈ or ˧˦˨	Rising falling
↓ Downstep		↗ Global rise	
↑ Upstep		↘ Global fall	

Index

Old English 150–54; *see also* History of English
opaque orthographies 174, 184; *see also* orthography
open class 58–59, 78–79
oral sound 14, 24
oral stop 16, 17, 24
orthography 11, 23, 155, 174–75, 178
outer circle 145–46; *see also* World Englishes

palatals 15, 18, 52
paradigm leveling 133
parts of speech 78–82
pharynx 12–15, 18,
phoneme 36, 38, 41–42, 48–49
phonetic environment 37, 40–43, 61
phonetic inventory 3, 141, 183
phonetics 3, 6, 23, 115–117
phonics 23, 43
phonographic 174, 178–79, 184; *see also* writing systems
phonological processes 44–45, 47
phonology 4, 6, 35, 40, 51, 117
phrasal semantics 103–104
phrase structure rules 82–83, 93–94, 98, 104
pidgins 138, 142, 143, 144
pitch 26–29, 67, 124
polysemy 101–102
Portuguese language 70, 127, 144
pragmatics 5–6, 105–106, 115
predicates 79, 87, 90, 103; intransitive predicates 104; transitive predicates 104
Prehistory of English 150; *see also* History of English
printing press 154, 157
prodrop languages 94

Q'anjob'al language 145
Quechua language 18

reduplication 67, 144–45, 147
reference 99–100
r-lessness 128–29; *see also* language discrimination
Romansch language 141–42
Russian language 116, 127

Sanskrit language 176–77
semantic roles 103–104
semantics 5–6, 98, 115

semilinguals 165; *see also* bilingualism misconceptions
sense 99
Singlish language 146–47; *see also* World Englishes
slang 116–18, 133
sociolinguistics 115, 118, 133, 135
soft palate 13–14
Spanish language 17, 22, 24–27, 38, 52, 63–64, 70–73, 119–20, 127, 131–32, 140–41, 145, 167–68, 183–85
speech acts 111
speech community 115, 119, 124, 164
spoken language 174–75
Sranan language 148–49; *see also* creoles
stress 26–31; primary stress 27, 37, 54, 66; secondary stress 27
stress timed languages 29–30
structural borrowing 141; *see also* borrowing
subject 87; subject drop 94
substrate language 142; *see also* pidgins
subtractive bilingualism 168, 171
superstrate language 142; *see also* pidgins
suppletion 68
suprasegmentals 26
Swahili language 24
syllabic writing system 181
syllables 48–51
syllable-timed languages 29–30
syntax 5–6, 76, 103, 115

Thai language 27, 29
Tibetan language 176–77
tone 29, 105, 147
transitional bilingual education 168–69; *see also* bilingual education
transparent orthographies 174, 183–84; *see also* orthography
tree diagrams 83–85
Turkish language 75, 131, 145
two-way immersion 169–70; *see also* bilingual education

unaspirated 36–38, 47, 140
upspeak 127; *see also* language discrimination

velum 13, 15–17, 20, 24
verbs 78–79, 103
vocal cords 12, 16, 46, 127–28
vocal fry 127; *see also* language discrimination

Printed in the United States
by Baker & Taylor Publisher Services